Application of
NURSING PROCESS and NURSING DIAGNOSIS:
An Interactive Text

Complimentary clinical reminder cards listing nursing diagnoses and outlining patient diagnostic statements are supplied in the back of this book.

Application of
NURSING PROCESS
and NURSING DIAGNOSIS:
An Interactive Text

MARILYNN E. DOENGES RN, BSN, MA, CS

Clinical Specialist
Adult Psychiatric/Mental Health Nursing
Private Practice
Instructor
Beth El College of Nursing
Colorado Springs, Colorado

MARY FRANCES MOORHOUSE RN, CCP, CCRN, CRRN

Nurse Consultant
TNT-RN Enterprises and Fortis Corporation
Colorado Springs, Colorado

with   Susan M. McCoy
       Editorial Associate

 F.A. DAVIS COMPANY • Philadelphia

Aquisitions editor: Robert G. Martone
Developmental editor: Susan McCoy
Production editor: Rose Gabbay
Cover design by Donald B. Freggens, Jr.

As new scientific information becomes available through basic and clinical research, recommended treatments and drug therapies undergo changes. The author(s) and publisher have done everything possible to make this book accurate, up to date, and in accord with accepted standards at the time of publication. The authors, editors, and publisher are not responsible for errors or omissions or for consequences from application of the book, and make no warranty, expressed or implied, in regard to the contents of the book. Any practice described in this book should be applied by the reader in accordance with professional standards of care used in regard to the unique circumstances that may apply in each situation. The reader is advised always to check product information (package inserts) for changes and new information regarding dose and contraindications before administering any drug. Caution is especially urged when using new or infrequently ordered drugs.

To our families, who support us in all that we do.

To our editor, Robert Martone, who coerced and hounded us to complete this project and who has marvelous ideas about what needs to be done.

To Susan McCoy, who is not only a superb design editor, but who clarified our thoughts and polished our words.

To the students of Beth El College of Nursing on clinical rotation for Mental Health Nursing at Cedar Springs Psychiatric Hospital, Spring, 1991, who challenged me to make nursing process and diagnosis understandable and provided me with valuable feedback.

To the rest of the F.A. Davis family, especially Herb Powell and Rose Gabbay, thanks for all your hard work in the production and completion of this project.

and last, but not least . . .

To our colleagues who are continuing to define and refine nursing process and nursing diagnosis, we hope this workbook will help students at all stages to clarify and apply these concepts.

Notes to the Educator

Nursing process is central to nursing actions in any setting. It is an efficient method of organizing thought processes for clinical decision-making and problem-solving when planning and delivering patient care. Although methods for streamlining the documentation of care in clinical settings have been proposed and, in some places, instituted, educational institutions must continue to instill in their students clinical decision-making skills rooted in the nursing process.

State and national accrediting agencies and national nursing organizations agree that patient/client care must be planned, evaluated, and documented. Although the format for the "care plan" may change over time, the activities reflected in the mechanics of care plan construction will still need to be performed and documented in the patient's permanent record to assure appropriate, cost-effective, and high quality care.

This text focuses on the nursing process and on how your students can use it effectively to enhance their nursing practice. By identifying the steps of the process clearly and concisely, it leads the student step by step, promoting an understanding of how the components fit together in a continuous cycle of thought and action.

Patient vignettes are presented to walk your students through the nursing process. The nurse's role of intervening to problem-solve, either independently or collaboratively with other health team members, is clearly identified throughout.

Chapter 1 presents an overview of the nursing process and its importance to daily practice. Chapter 2 provides information and a tool for doing a nursing assessment to gather accurate data and create the patient database.

Chapter 3 discusses problem identification and the use of nursing diagnoses to write the patient diagnostic statement.

In Chapter 4, goal setting, the selection of patient outcomes, and nursing actions/interventions are discussed in connection with development of the plan of care.

Chapter 5 presents information about the validation and implementation of the plan of care. In Chapter 6 evaluation and modification of the plan are discussed to show how the process is completed.

The importance and necessity of documenting the nursing process is interwoven throughout the book. A variety of documentation models are presented in Chapter 7 to provide an opportunity for the student to practice this skill and to promote flexibility within multiple healthcare settings. To further enhance use of the nursing process, the list of NANDA-approved nursing diagnoses has been included in Appendix A. The related/risk factors and defining characteristics have been listed to aid selection of the appropriate nursing diagnosis label, and to develop diagnostic statements quickly, confidently, and accurately.

This text has been designed to provide a highly interactive, hands-on experience with the nursing process. Tearout pages for independent learning are an important feature of this text, providing an opportunity for practical application and mastery of the nursing process. It is our hope that the interactive features of this book will assist the learner in making an effective transition from the classroom to any clinical setting.

Marilynn E. Doenges
Mary Frances Moorhouse

Acknowledgments

To Sally Olds, RN, MS

    Associate Professor
    Beth El College of Nursing
    Colorado Springs, Colorado
    whose input and critique enabled us to make this project more useful to
    students at all stages. Thank you.

To Barbara Mahoney, RN, MA, CS

    Clinical Specialist Psychiatric Nurse
    Private Practice
    Colorado Springs, Colorado

To Paladin Productions

    whose computer talents clarified our ideas and made them visible.

Contents

Practice Activities and Work Pages

EVALUATION

DOCUMENTATION

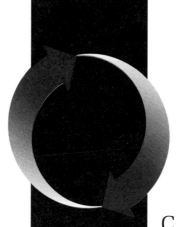

CHAPTER 1

The Nursing Process: Delivering Quality Care

THE NURSING PROFESSION

Nursing is both a science and an art, and as such, it is concerned with the physical, psychologic, sociologic, cultural, and spiritual concerns of the individual. The science of nursing is based on a broad theoretical framework, while its art is dependent upon the caring skills and abilities of the individual nurse. The importance of the nurse within the healthcare system is being recognized in many positive ways, and the profession of nursing is itself acknowledging the need for its practitioners to be professional and accountable.

In its early developmental years, nursing did not seek or have the means to control its own practice. Florence Nightingale, in discussing the nature of nursing, observed that "nursing has been limited to signify little more than the administration of medicines and the application of poultices" (Nightingale, 1859). While this societal attitude has persisted into the present, the nursing profession has been working to define what it is that uniquely characterizes

1

what nurses do that other healthcare providers do not do, and to identify nursing's body of professional knowledge.

Thus, barely a century after Miss Nightingale noted that "the very elements of nursing are all but unknown," the American Nurses Association developed the ANA *Social Policy Statement* defining nursing as "the diagnosis and treatment of human responses to actual and potential health problems." In the modern world of nursing, therefore, human responses are the phenomena of concern for nurses.

THE NURSING PROCESS

The nursing profession has identified a problem-solving process that "combines the most desirable elements of the art of nursing with the most relevant elements of systems theory, using the scientific method" (Shore, 1988).

This Nursing Process was introduced in the 1950s as a three-step process of *assessment, planning,* and *evaluation* based on the scientific method of observing, measuring, gathering data, and analyzing the findings. Years of study, use, and refinement have led nurses to expand the nursing process to five concrete steps which provide an efficient method of organizing thought processes for clinical decision-making, problem-solving, and the delivery of higher-quality, individualized patient care. Box 1–1 shows the steps and their order. These five steps are central to nursing actions in any setting. The nursing process is now included in the conceptual framework of most nursing curricula and is accepted as part of the legal definition of nursing in the Nurse Practice Acts of many states.

According to the steps of the nursing process, when a patient enters the healthcare system, the nurse collects data, identifies problems/needs (nursing diagnoses), establishes goals, identifies outcomes, and chooses nursing interventions to achieve these outcomes and goals. Finally, after these interventions have been carried out, the nurse evaluates the effectiveness of the plan of care in reaching the desired outcomes and goals to determine whether or not the problems have been resolved and the patient is ready to leave the system. If the identified problems *remain* unresolved, further assessment, additional

DEFINITION OF
NURSING PROCESS

The Nursing Process is a five-step process:

1. Nursing Assessment

2. Problem Identification/ Analysis (nursing diagnosis)

3. Planning

4. Implementation

5. Evaluation

The Nursing Process provides an orderly, logical problem-solving approach for administering nursing care so that the patient's needs for such care are met comprehensively and effectively.

BOX 1–1 STEPS OF THE NURSING PROCESS

The nursing process consists of five specific steps or "phases":

1. **Assessment:** A systematic collection of data relating to patients
2. **Problem Identification:** Analysis of data to identify the patient's problems and needs
3. **Planning:** Setting goals, identifying outcomes, and choosing interventions to create a plan of care to treat the problems and needs identified in the previous step
4. **Implementation:** Putting the plan of care into action
5. **Evaluation:** Assessing the effectiveness of the plan and changing the plan if indicated

problem identification, alteration of outcomes and goals, and/or changes of interventions are required.

Although we use the terms *assessment, problem identification, planning, implementation,* and *evaluation* as separate, progressive steps, in reality they are interrelated elements. Together, these elements form a continuous circle of thought and action, which recycles throughout the patient's contact with the healthcare system. Figure 1–1 gives some idea of how this cycling process works. You can see that the nursing process combines all of the skills of critical thinking and creates a method of active problem-solving that is both dynamic and cyclic.

THE USE OF THE NURSING PROCESS

There are many advantages to the use of the nursing process:

- The nursing process provides a framework within which the individual needs of the patient, the patient's family, and the community can be met.
- The steps of the nursing process focus the nurse's attention on the "individual" human responses of a patient/group to a given medical situation, resulting in a holistic plan of care addressing these specific problems/needs.
- The nursing process provides an organized, systematic method of problem-solving, minimizing dangerous errors or omissions in caregiving and avoiding time-consuming repetition in care and documentation.
- The use of the nursing process promotes the active involvement of the patient in his or her own health care, enhancing consumer satisfaction. Such participation increases the patient's sense of control over what is happening to him or her, stimulates problem-solving, and promotes personal responsibility . . . all of which strengthen the patient's commitment to achieving identified goals.

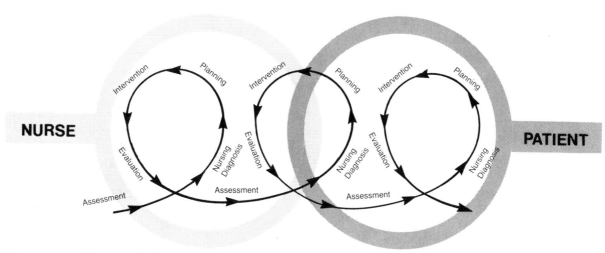

Figure 1–1. Diagram of the nursing process. The steps of the nursing process are interrelated, forming a continuous circle of thought and action that is both dynamic and cyclic.

- The use of the nursing process enables you as a nurse to have more control over your own practice. This enhances the opportunity for you to use your knowledge, expertise, and intuition constructively and dynamically to increase the likelihood of a successful patient outcome. This, in turn, promotes greater job satisfaction and professional growth.
- The use of the nursing process provides a common language for practice, unifying the nursing profession. Using a system that clearly communicates the plan of care to coworkers and patients enhances continuity of care, promotes achievement of patient goals, aids in the development of nursing standards, and provides a vehicle for evaluation.
- The use of the nursing process provides a means of assessing nursing's economic contribution to patient care. The nursing process supplies a vehicle for the quantitative and qualitative measurement of nursing care that meets the goal of cost effectiveness and still promotes holistic care.

HOW THE NURSING PROCESS WORKS

The scientific method of problem-solving introduced in the previous section is used almost instinctively by most people, without conscious awareness, as noted in Box 1–2. Since the nursing process is based on this method, it may well seem somewhat familiar. You will only need to learn the new format required by the nursing process, rather than having to think about each step (assessment, problem identification, planning, implementation, and evaluation) in an entirely new way.

To effectively use the nursing process, there are fundamental abilities which the nurse must possess and be able to apply. Particularly important is a thorough knowledge of science and theory—not only as applied in nursing, but also as applied in other related disciplines such as medicine and psychology. Creativity is needed in the application of nursing knowledge, as well as adaptability in handling change and the many unexpected happenings which

---

BOX 1–2 PROBLEM SOLVING: EVERYDAY USE OF THE NURSING PROCESS

You have celebrated completion of your semester finals with a spicy curry dinner. You awaken during the night with a burning sensation in the center of your chest. You are young and in good health and note no other symptoms (assessment). You decide that your pain is the result of the spicy food you have eaten (problem identification). You then determine that you need to relieve the discomfort before you will be able to return to sleep (planning). You take an antacid liquid (implementation). Within a few moments, you note the burning is relieved, and you return to bed and sleep (evaluation).

This is a process you routinely use to solve problems in your own life that can be readily applied to patient care situations.

occur. As a nurse, you must make a commitment to practice your profession in the best possible way, trusting in yourself and your ability to do your job well and displaying the necessary leadership to organize and supervise as your position requires. In addition, intelligence, well-developed interpersonal skills, and competent technical skills are essential.

> **For example:** A patient's irritable behavior could be a sign of anger or arise from a sense of helplessness regarding life events. However, it could also be the result of low blood sugar or the effects of excessive caffeine intake. A single behavior may have varied causes. It is important that your nursing assessment skills identify the underlying etiology.

In addition to these abilities, there are several fundamental beliefs (Box 1–3) that, when actualized by the nurse, provide guidance for the application of the nursing process and enhance the quality of nursing care.

Effective use of the nursing process is a product of your efforts and thoughts, and its documentation meets the Standards of Nursing Practice set forth by the American Nurses Association (Table 1–1). With the ultimate goal of quality health care, the effective use of the nursing process will result in a viable nursing-care system that is recognized and accepted as nursing's body of knowledge and that can be shared with other healthcare professionals.

SUMMARY

In using the nursing process to administer nursing care to patients, the nursing profession has identified a body of knowledge that contributes to the prevention of illness as well as to the maintenance and/or restoration of the patient's health (or relief of pain and discomfort when a return to health is not possible). The nursing process is the basis of all nursing actions and is the essence of nursing. It can be applied in any healthcare or educational setting, in any theoretical or conceptual framework, and within the context of any nursing philosophy. The process is flexible and yet sufficiently structured so as to provide the base for nursing actions.

Table 1–1 ANA STANDARDS OF PRACTICE

  I. The collection of data about the health status of the client/patient is systematic and continuous. The data are accessible, communicated, and recorded.
 II. Nursing diagnoses are derived from health status data.
III. The plan of nursing care includes goals derived from the nursing diagnoses.
 IV. The plan of nursing care includes the priorities and the prescribed nursing approaches or measures to achieve the goals derived from the nursing diagnoses.
  V. Nursing actions provide for client/patient participation and health promotion, maintenance, and restoration.
 VI. Nursing actions assist the client/patient to maximize his or her health capabilities.
VII. The client's/patient's progress or lack of progress toward goal achievement is determined by the client/patient and the nurse.
VIII. The client's/patient's progress or lack of progress toward goal achievement directs reassessment, reordering of priorities, new goal setting, and revision of the plan of nursing care.

Reproduced with the permission of ANA from Standards of Nursing Practice, ANA, 1973.

> ### BOX 1–3 FUNDAMENTAL PHILOSOPHICAL BELIEFS IN NURSING
>
> There are several fundamental philosophical beliefs which are essential to the practice of nursing and which need to be kept in mind when using the nursing process:
>
> - The patient is a human being who has worth and dignity.
> - There are basic human needs such as those described in Maslow's Hierarchy (see Chapter 2) which must be met. When they are not met, problems arise that may require intervention by another person until the individual can resume responsibility for self.
> - Patients have a right to quality health and nursing care delivered with interest, compassion, and competence and focused on wellness and prevention.
> - The therapeutic nurse-patient relationship is important in this process.

The following chapters will identify, discuss, and clarify each step of the nursing process, providing information to reinforce your understanding and opportunities to apply your knowledge by means of Practice Activities and a Work Page at the end of each chapter. Six patients will be helping you in your learning process by sharing their personal experiences:

- Robert is a 72-year-old man with pneumonia.
- Jennifer is a 3-year-old child with a chronic ear infection.
- Sally is a 30-year-old woman who is pregnant and experiencing beginning labor.
- Mike, a 20-year-old man, has suffered multiple injuries in a motorcycle accident.
- Donald, a 46-year-old man, is being treated for depression.
- Martha, a 52-year-old woman, has had her gallbladder removed.

Their ongoing case histories will provide many clinical examples throughout the text.

WORK PAGE: Chapter One

1. The American Nurses Association has defined nursing as: _____

   _____

2. My own definition of nursing is: _____

   _____

3. The *ANA Social Policy Statement* defines the phenomena of concern for nurses as: _____

   _____

4. The definition of Nursing Process is: _____

   _____

5. List and describe the five steps of the Nursing Process:

   a. _____

   b. _____

   c. _____

   d. _____

   e. _____

6. Choose three advantages of using the Nursing Process that you think are the most important:

   a. _____

   b. _____

   c. _____

7. Identify three of the fundamental philosophical assumptions basic to decision-making within the

   Nursing Process: _____

   _____

   _____

8. Identify the steps of the Nursing Process by numbering the appropriate activity in the following
   vignette:
   1 = Assessment;   2 = Problem identification;   3 = Planning;   4 = Implementation;   and
   5 = Evaluation.

Vignette: Robert, a 72-year-old male, is admitted with pneumonia. _____

He reports that this is his second episode in 6 months. _____

Temperature is 101°F, skin hot and flushed. _____

He complains of frequent, hacking cough with moderate amount of thick greenish mucus. _____

Auscultation of the chest reveals scattered rhonchi throughout. _____

His mucous membranes are pale, and his lips are dry and cracked. _____

You determine that Robert has an ineffective airway clearance, a fluid volume deficit, and a knowledge deficit that will require teaching to promote adequate self-care and to prevent recurrence. _____

You establish the following outcomes:

- Expectorates secretions completely with breath sounds clear and respiration noiseless.

  _____

- Demonstrates adequate fluid balance with moist mucous membranes and loose respiratory secretions. _____

- Verbalizes understanding of cause of condition and therapeutic regimen. _____

You decide to set up a regular schedule for respiratory activities and fluid replacement. _____

In addition, you formulate a teaching plan to cover the identified concerns for self-care and illness prevention. _____

You provide a tube of petroleum jelly for Robert to use on his lips. _____

Every 2 hours you visit Robert to encourage him to deep-breathe, cough, change his position, and drink a glass of fluid of his choice. _____

You use this time to discuss avoidance of crowds and individuals with upper respiratory infections and recommend continuing the treatment plan after discharge. _____

The following day, Robert's skin is no longer hot and flushed, temperature is 99°F, secretions are loose and readily expectorated, and breath sounds are clearing. _____

Robert's lips and oral mucous membranes are moist. _____

He is able to explain in his own words how to care for himself and how to prevent pneu-

monia. _____

You decide that the current treatment plan is achieving the identified outcomes and to continue

the plan as written. _____

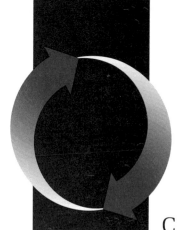

CHAPTER 2

The Assessment Phase: Developing the Patient Database

ANA Standard 1: The collection of data about the health status of the client/ patient is systematic and continuous. The data are accessible, communicated, and recorded.

THE PATIENT DATABASE

ASSESSMENT—the first step of the Nursing Process, during which data are collected.

PATIENT DATABASE —the compilation of data collected about a patient; it consists of the nursing history, physical examination, and results of the diagnostic studies.

SUBJECTIVE DATA— what the patient reports, believes, or feels.

OBJECTIVE DATA— what can be observed, for example, vital signs, behaviors, diagnostic studies.

The **ASSESSMENT** phase of the Nursing Process involves three basic activities: (1) systematically gathering data, (2) sorting and organizing the data collected, and (3) documenting (in a methodical way) the information that has been obtained. Using a number of techniques, the nurse focuses on eliciting a profile of the patient that will allow her or him to identify nursing diagnoses, plan care, implement interventions, and evaluate outcomes which are individualized for that patient's unique combination of needs. This profile is called the **PATIENT DATABASE**, and it serves as the fundamental pool of knowledge about the patient from which all other phases of the Nursing Process proceed.

The patient database supplies a sense of the patient's overall health status. It is a combination of data gathered from the history-taking interview (a method of obtaining **SUBJECTIVE** information by talking with the patient and/ or significant other(s) and listening to their responses); objective information from observing nonverbal behaviors and performing the physical assessment (a "hands-on" means of obtaining **OBJECTIVE** information using a systems, head-to-toe, or patient needs–based approach); and data gathered from the results of laboratory/diagnostic studies.

Because consistency is important, the same data collection model should be used for both history-taking and the physical assessment, whether that model is a nursing framework, a systems approach, a head-to-toe approach, or a combination approach defined by your own agency. Frequently, these two activities are combined into one interactive process in which physical data are gathered while interview questions are asked.

Framework for Data Collection

There are several nursing models which may be used to guide the nurse in data collection. Three of those most commonly used are shown in Table 2–1: Doenges and Moorhouse's Diagnostic Divisions, Gordon's Functional Health Patterns, and NANDA's Human Response Patterns.

The use of a nursing model as a framework (rather than a body systems or head-to-toe approach) has the advantage of facilitating collection of the data needed to identify and validate nursing diagnoses as opposed to medical diagnoses. A framework such as the Assessment Tool shown in Appendix B limits repetitive collection of medical data, and focuses data collection on the nurse's phenomena of concern: the physiologic, sociocultural, psychologic, developmental, and environmental factors that are affecting the patient.

The Interview Process

Information in the patient database is obtained both from the patient and from family members/significant others (as appropriate) through conversation and by observation during a structured interview. The nursing interview may take place over several contact sessions, but each contact should yield information, verify information already gathered, or clarify data. A well-conducted interview can be the first step in establishing a beneficial nurse/patient relationship and the rapport needed for good communication.

However, the interview is not merely the routine completion of the items

Table 2–1 **COMPARISON OF NURSING MODELS FOR DATA COLLECTION**

DIAGNOSTIC DIVISIONS (DOENGES AND MOORHOUSE, 1991)	FUNCTIONAL HEALTH PATTERNS (GORDON, 1987)	HUMAN RESPONSE PATTERNS (NANDA, 1990)
ACTIVITY/REST: Ability to engage in necessary/desired activities of life (work and leisure), and to obtain sleep/rest.	**HEALTH PERCEPTION/ HEALTH MANAGEMENT:** Client's perception of general health status and well-being. Adherence to preventative health practices.	**CHOOSING:** To select between alternatives; the action of selecting or exercising preference in regard to a matter in which one is a free agent; to determine in favor of a course; to decide in accordance with inclinations.
CIRCULATION: Ability to transport oxygen and nutrients necessary to meet cellular needs.	**NUTRITIONAL/METABOLIC:** Patterns of food and fluid intake, fluid and electrolyte balance, general ability to heal.	**COMMUNICATING:** To converse; to impart, confer or transmit thoughts, feelings or information, internally or externally, verbally or nonverbally.
EGO INTEGRITY: Ability to develop and use skills and behaviors to integrate and manage life experiences.	**ELIMINATION:** Patterns of excretory function (bowel, bladder and skin), and client's perception.	**EXCHANGING:** To give, relinquish or lose something while receiving something in return; the substitution of one element for another; the reciprocal act of giving and receiving.
ELIMINATION: Ability to excrete waste products.	**ACTIVITY/EXERCISE:** Pattern of exercise, activity, leisure, recreation, and ADLs, factors that interfere with desired or expected individual pattern.	
FOOD/FLUID: Ability to maintain intake of and utilize nutrients and liquids to meet physiologic needs.		**FEELING:** To experience, a consciousness, sensation, apprehension or sense; to be consciously or emotionally affected by a fact, event or state.
HYGIENE: Ability to perform activities of daily living.	**COGNITIVE/PERCEPTUAL:** Adequacy of sensory modes, such as vision, hearing, taste, touch, smell, pain perception, cognitive functional abilities.	**KNOWING:** To recognize or acknowledge a thing or a person; to be familiar with by experience or through information or report; to be cognizant of something through observation, inquiry or information; to be conversant with a body of facts, principles, or methods of action; to understand.
NEUROSENSORY: Ability to perceive, integrate, and respond to internal and external cues.		
PAIN/COMFORT: Ability to control internal/external environment to maintain comfort.	**SLEEP/REST:** Patterns of sleep and rest-relaxation periods during twenty-four hour day, as well as quality and quantity.	
RESPIRATION: Ability to provide and utilize oxygen to meet physiologic needs.	**SELF-PERCEPTION/SELF- CONCEPT:** Individual's attitudes about self, perception of abilities, body image, identity, general sense of worth and emotional patterns.	**MOVING:** To change the place or position of the body or any member of the body; to put and/or keep in motion; to provoke an excretion or discharge; the urge to action or to do something; to take action.
SAFETY: Ability to provide safe, growth promoting environment.		
SEXUALITY: (Component of Ego Integrity and Social Interaction) Ability to meet requirements/characteristics of male/female role.		
SOCIAL INTERACTION: Ability to establish and maintain relationships.	**ROLE/RELATIONSHIP:** Client's perception of major roles and responsibilities in current life situation.	**PERCEIVING:** To apprehend with the mind; to become
TEACHING/LEARNING: Ability to incorporate and use information to achieve healthy lifestyle/optimal wellness.	**SEXUALITY/ REPRODUCTIVE:** Client's perceived satisfaction or dissatisfaction with sexuality. Reproductive stage and pattern.	

(Continued)

Table 2–1 **COMPARISON OF NURSING MODELS FOR** (Continued)
DATA COLLECTION

DIAGNOSTIC DIVISIONS (DOENGES AND MOORHOUSE, 1991)	FUNCTIONAL HEALTH PATTERNS (GORDON, 1987)	HUMAN RESPONSE PATTERNS (NANDA, 1990)
	COPING/STRESS TOLERANCE: General coping pattern, stress tolerance, support systems, and perceived ability to control and manage situations. **VALUE/BELIEF:** Values, goals, or beliefs that guide choices or decisions.	aware of by the senses; to apprehend what is not open or present to observation; to take fully or adequately. **RELATING:** To connect, to establish a link between, to stand in some association to another thing, person or place; to be borne or thrust in between things. **VALUING:** To be concerned about, to care about the worth or worthiness, the relative status of a thing, or the estimate in which it is held, according to its real or supposed worth, usefulness, or importance; one's opinion of or liking for a person or thing; to equate in importance.

BOX 2–1 SUBJECTIVE VS. OBJECTIVE DATA

Subjective data are what the patient/significant other(s) say reflecting their own thoughts, feelings, and perceptions:

"My hip hurts."

"I'm worried about surgery."

"She didn't sleep well."

"I can't give my husband a shot."

"I haven't had a bowel movement for 3 days."

"I don't think I'll ever get better."

"I can't walk that far."

"I don't know what to do."

"His usual weight is 160 pounds."

Objective data are observable and measurable and include information gathered during the physical assessment and diagnostic studies:

Restless/agitated

Temperature 99.2°F

Old surgical scar

Flabby muscle tone

Hgb 12.4

Cardiac murmur

Putrid odor

Bloody vomitus

Facial grimacing

Glucose 107

on a form by whoever is available. Rather, it is a tool of communication that permits an *exchange* of information, a process which produces a level of understanding higher than that which either person could achieve alone. The nursing interview thus has a specific purpose: the collection of a set of specific data (information) that are obtained from the patient and/or significant other(s) through both conversation (subjective data) and observation (objective data). Box 2–1 provides some examples to clarify the distinction between these two forms of data. Now, take a few moments to work through Practice Activity 2–1.

Clearly, more than simply exchanging and processing data is sought. Nonverbal communication is as important as the patient's choice of words in providing the data. The ability to collect data meaningful to the patient's health concerns depends heavily on the nurse's own knowledge base; the choice and sequence of questions; and the ability to give meaning to the patient's responses, integrate the data gathered, and prioritize the resulting information. The nurse's knowledge, understanding, and insight into the nature and behavior of the patient are essential elements as well.

Now, take a few more moments and read through Box 2–2, which identifies ten key elements for a successful interview. As you begin to work with these techniques, you will see that they provide an opportunity for the patient to use descriptive terms and to explain more fully the meaning of an answer. You will want to keep these tips in mind as you complete the practice activities in this chapter.

The question is the major tool you will use to obtain information, as discussed in Box 2–3. How you phrase the question is a skill that is important in obtaining the desired results and getting the information necessary to make nursing diagnoses that will promote the best outcome for the patient. However, be aware that even with a properly phrased question, there will be times when the answer you are seeking will not be given. It is important to remember, too, that the patient has the right to refuse to answer any question at all, no matter how reasonably phrased. Box 2–4 highlights some questioning strategies that are generally ineffective in eliciting information from patients.

THE NURSING INTERVIEW: QUESTIONING AND LISTENING

The patient's **MEDICAL DIAGNOSIS** can provide a starting point for the nursing interview. The nurse's knowledge about the anatomy and physiology of the disease condition helps in the choice and prioritizing of questions. Remember, though, that the *results* of this focused interview process will point to the human responses to illness which are the phenomena of nursing concern, and therefore, to the development of *nursing* (rather than medical) diagnoses. For example, although you will ask Robert about the signs and symptoms associated with his pneumonia, your focus will be:

- How does his shortness of breath affect his ability to care for himself?
- Have the coughing episodes resulted in chest wall pain or loss of sleep?
- Has his appetite been affected by his frequent expectoration of purulent mucus?
- How does he protect others from transmission of infection?

Remember:

- The **BETTER YOU ARE PREPARED** for the interview, the better your chances of asking something revealing that provides new insights about the patient, which in turn will help you to ask more pertinent questions.

- The **BETTER LISTENER YOU ARE**, the better your chance of hearing something meaningful in the patient's responses.

- The **MORE PERCEPTIVE YOU ARE**, the better your chances of seeing new relationships among the data collected.

MEDICAL DIAGNOSIS
— illnesses/conditions for which treatment is directed by a licensed physician; medical diagnoses focus on correction/prevention of the pathology of specific organs/body systems.

PRACTICE ACTIVITY 2-1

DETERMINING TYPES OF DATA

1. Identify Subjective (S) versus Objective (O) data:

   _____ Skin cool/damp

   _____ Sputum pale yellow

   _____ Allergic to eggs and sulfa

   _____ Pitting edema of feet and ankles

   _____ Usually voids three times per day

   _____ Chest pain lasting 15 minutes

2. Match the technique in column A to the statements in column B:

   Column A

   a. Open-ended question

   b. Hypothetical question

   c. Reflection

   d. Closed-ended question

   e. Leading question

   Column B

   _____ The next time this comes up, what would you do to handle it?

   _____ That feeling in your chest, can you describe it more fully?

   _____ Do you use alcohol regularly?

   _____ Is there something you would like to talk about?

   _____ You're feeling better today, aren't you?

3. Rewrite the following as open-ended questions:

   a. You felt like crying, didn't you?

   b. You're in pain again?

   c. Do you want to change occupations?

   d. Since your doctor has talked with you, you don't have any questions, do you?

   e. Did you eat lunch?

In addition, the nurse needs to keep an open mind and pay attention to clues which may identify other areas requiring investigation.

The Patient History

The period of time devoted to obtaining a patient history is well spent, since it is a significant factor in saving time later on in the delivery of any healthcare services to patients and/or significant other(s). Insufficient time allocated to obtaining the patient history can result in failure to obtain critical information. Failure to obtain data may, in turn, create a climate of distrust and could significantly add to the length and cost of the patient's care.

The history is more than simply recording information. The nurse must review the data, organize and determine the relevance of each item (value the data), and document the facts. The quality of a history improves with the nurse's knowledge and experience with the history-taking process. Although such assessments are often lengthy and time-consuming in the beginning, more time is eventually saved by avoiding the necessity to retrace steps, correct misinformation, and undo actions. With practice, the time required for this activity will decrease.

Guidelines for History-taking

LISTEN CAREFULLY

Be a good listener: The nurse needs to listen attentively to what the individual is saying. Listen for whole thoughts and ideas, not merely for isolated facts. Facts may not be as important as the ideas that bind them together. For example, a diabetic patient may tell you, "Yes, I understand my diet. I am on a 2500-calorie-a-day exchange diet and take 100 units of NPH insulin daily," but the patient's tone of voice, facial expression, and body language communicate the idea that the individual does not accept his diabetes and may not be following his diet closely. This nonverbal communication needs to be validated by asking something like: "You seem to have a lack of enthusiasm as you tell me about your diet and insulin. What is that about?"

ACTIVE LISTENING

Use skills of active listening, silence, and acceptance to provide ample time for the person to respond: Give your full attention to the interview and do not interrupt. Save your own comments until the speaker is completely finished. Finally, ask related questions to stimulate the individual's memory if blocks occur.

Active listening is a process of validation, by feeding back, to the patient, words and feelings that you hear.

OBJECTIVITY

Be as objective as possible: Identify only the patient's and/or significant others' contributions in this history, and do not try to interpret the data at this point. Record subjective data from the patient/significant other(s) just as it was stated during the interview. Failure to do so may confuse the issue.

However, lengthy responses may need to be paraphrased within the same constraints. The nurse's initial responsibility is to observe, collect, and record data without drawing conclusions or making judgments/assumptions. A crucial factor in the process of data collection is the nurse's own self-awareness in the interaction, since one's own perceptions, judgments, and assumptions can easily color the assessment findings unless they are recognized. We all have a responsibility to know and minimize the impact of our own biases and beliefs on the data gathered and the conclusions drawn from them.

BOX 2-2   ELEMENTS OF A SUCCESSFUL INTERVIEW

A successful interview has **10 key elements:** (1) a clear sense of the underlying purpose for conducting the interview, (2) preliminary or background research before the interview begins, (3) a formal request of the interviewee to conduct the interview, (4) sound interviewing strategy, (5) effective use of icebreakers, (6) smoothly addressing the business of the interview, (7) good rapport between nurse and patient, (8) sensitivity to the patient's needs during the interview process, (9) adequate time for recovery following discussion of sensitive areas, and (10) definitive closure of the interview.

1. **Underlying purpose:** Stated specifically, the information to be gathered during the interview will be used in formulating the plan of care. This provides guidance in asking as well as answering questions, especially when areas that appear to be unrelated to the current situation may need to be pursued.

2. **Preliminary research:** Investigate the patient's and the patient's family's current and previous situation. Resources such as prior admission records and other health team members can be used. Notes can be made to identify key points. This research generates questions that should be written down so they are not lost. When the point of asking questions in the interview is reached, you will know most of the areas that need to be addressed. The end result of the interview is dependent on what is put into it.

3. **Request to conduct the interview:** Formally requesting the interview of the interviewee is courteous and can clearly promote a positive interaction. You identify yourself to the patient and explain precisely the purpose of collecting the data and how that data will be used. Together, a time is set for the interview, giving consideration to the needs/severity of the patient's condition and availability of significant others to allow for time to prepare for the interview when possible. Your approach and attitude are important in helping the patient to be comfortable and to understand the importance of the interview. "Mr. Jones, I would like to ask you some questions about yourself and your illness, so that together we may plan your care," is a much more positive approach than, "I need to know your history." The first approach not only sells the interview but stimulates the patient's thinking. The result is a more productive interview.

4. **Interview strategy:** Cover the details of the interview in accordance with the definition of its purpose. Preparation and planning give a sense of security and a plan to fall back on if things go slowly or unexpectedly wrong. This also allows a comfortable departure from the plan when conversation takes an unexplored path into productive channels. A new twist and a refreshing insight are the gold nuggets of interviewing, leading to information that otherwise might not have been remembered or shared.

5. **Icebreakers:** Icebreakers are the words and phrases which can help to put the patient at ease, set the stage, and promote a relaxed situation. How the icebreakers are used during the first few minutes may

(Continued)

BOX 2-2   ELEMENTS OF A SUCCESSFUL INTERVIEW (*Continued*)

determine how and if the interview proceeds. Within these first minutes of the interview session, you, the patient, and/or significant other(s) will make important decisions concerning the future of this relationship. During these minutes, the patient, and/or significant other(s) are making judgments about you, that is, that you are sincere, trustworthy, sensitive, professionally competent, or not. The icebreakers used at the beginning of the interview have vital importance in answering these questions. It is the first bond of human communication and trust in this new relationship. When you sit down and appear relaxed and interested, this goal is more readily achieved. Some examples of icebreakers which might be used are the acknowledgment of what you know and see: "You've been admitted for surgery." or "You're concerned about coming to the hospital." A comment about the weather, "We certainly have been having a lot of rain," may put the patient at ease. Offering something to drink, if allowed, and asking the patient how he or she prefers to be addressed will also serve to promote an atmosphere of relaxation.

6. **Business:** Get to the business at hand. Ask the questions that were previously determined, using terminology the patient understands. Listen then for answers and clues that will lead to other questions that may not have been anticipated. The relaxed informality, which has been achieved before, continues through this phase. Do not expect insights immediately, as they usually come with time, increased comfort level, and trust.

7. **Rapport:** Participants usually settle down as the conversation proceeds. Call the participants by name, and monitor reactions to questions. Be careful not to bore or intimidate them with embarrassing questions. It is important to know when to shift gears, speed up, or slow down; or when to ask more challenging questions. Do not hurry the interview, and maintain eye contact as appropriate based on cultural belief systems. For instance, some Asian and Native American cultures believe it is disrespectful to make eye contact.

8. **Sensitivity:** It may be necessary to ask questions about issues which involve sensitive areas for the patient. Such questions may be perceived as threatening in nature. For example, questions about sexuality, lifestyle, or behaviors which may bring out the possibility of sexually transmitted diseases (STDs), including HIV and AIDS. It is important for the nurse to proceed gently toward these sensitive areas. Be alert to verbal/nonverbal cues that may indicate that the area of discussion is particularly sensitive for the individual. Ceasing exploration at this point demonstrates respect for the individual's rights/privacy and can enhance the trust between you and the patient/significant other.

9. **Recovery:** Recover the rapport. If the sensitive areas have been approached slowly, the recovery period should be fairly easy to accomplish. Warmth and caring evidenced by a smile and a touch of the hand are helpful.

(Continued)

BOX 2-2   ELEMENTS OF A SUCCESSFUL INTERVIEW (Continued)

10. **Closure:** Conclude the interview by summarizing the highlights of the interview and leave the door open for further communication. An important way to do this is to ask the patient if he or she has anything else to add or any questions to ask of you.

BOX 2-3   EFFECTIVE DATA COLLECTION TECHNIQUES

- **Open-ended questions** allow maximum freedom for the patient to respond in his or her own way; impose no limitations on how the question may be answered; and can produce considerable information, such as, "How do you feel about your new medications?" or "Explain the injection techniques to me."
- **Hypothetical questions** pose a situation and ask the patient how it might be handled. You can learn whether the patient has accurate information and can think about how a similar situation might be handled. For example, "What would you do if you noticed a rash on your body?" or "What would you do if you felt dizzy?" These questions may be very useful in determining the extent to which the patient has learned previously presented material.
- **Reflecting or "mirroring" responses** are useful techniques in getting at underlying meanings that might not be verbalized clearly. The patient might say, "Some days I'd like to throw this needle out the window." A mirror response might be, "You feel angry about the needle?" Now the patient is encouraged to verbalize what she or he is actually angry about. This response is nonevaluative and nonthreatening.
- **Focusing** shows the patient that you are attending to what is being said and consists of eye contact (within cultural limits), body posture, and verbal responses. The message is, "Tell me more about that."
- **Giving broad openings** encourages the patient to take the initiative about what is to be talked about: "Where would you like to begin?"
- **Offering general leads** encourages the patient to continue: ". . . and then?"
- **Exploring** pursues a topic in more detail: "Would you describe it more fully?"
- **Verbalizing the implied** gives voice to what has been suggested; for instance, the patient says, "It's no use taking this medicine anymore." You respond, "You're concerned that it isn't making a difference for you?"
- **Encouraging evaluation** helps the patient to consider the quality of his or her own experience, such as: "How does that seem to you?"

MANAGEABLE DETAIL

Keep the amount of detail manageable: The data collected about the patient and/or significant other(s) contain a vast amount of information, some of which may be repetitious. This in turn may suggest a direction which has value for eliciting new/different information that was not recalled or volunteered previously.

Enough material needs to be noted in the history so that as complete a picture as possible is presented, and yet not so much that the information won't be read or used. "Necessary" information includes all data (positive and negative) that are relevant to the situation. Some description is usually needed to make the data more meaningful. For example, simply recording "cough" is not as informative as recording "cough productive, yellow, large amount."

SEQUENCE INFORMATION

Order is imperative: Develop and use an information-gathering form that facilitates finding information and that aids in problem identification and the choice of nursing diagnoses. In addition, present the current health problem in chronological order and include relevant events from the past. It is also useful to express topics in a uniform manner. For example, expressing the *age* at which events/illnesses/surgery occurred instead of the year events occurred: "age 67" versus "born in 1923"; or "hysterectomy, age 35" versus "hysterectomy, 1968."

DOCUMENT CLEARLY

Write legibly: This improves comprehension and the ability to communicate findings. It decreases the chance of misunderstanding, thus saving time for you as well as other healthcare professionals who rely on your records.

RECORD DATA IN A TIMELY WAY

Write the history as soon as possible after gathering the information: This makes the data more accurate, for the longer you wait to record, the more the data and specific details will fade away. Data not written are data lost.

PHYSICAL ASSESSMENT: THE HANDS-ON PHASE

The nurse performs the physical assessment for purposes of gathering objective information, and also as a screening device. For the data collected during the physical assessment to be meaningful, the nurse needs to know the normal physical and emotional characteristics of human beings sufficiently well enough to be able to recognize deviations.

Focus and Preparation

In order to gain as much information as possible from this assessment procedure, approach the patient with a positive, sincere attitude. Such an

---

BOX 2–4 GENERALLY INEFFECTIVE DATA COLLECTION TECHNIQUES

- **Closed-ended questions** (such as "Why?") which allow little or no freedom in choosing a response, such as, "Do you take your medicine?" (patient responds "No") or "How long have you been taking insulin?" (patient responds "3 years"). Typically there are only one or two possible answers to the question. The interviewer remains in close control over the interview because of the rigid structure. Although the closed-ended question may be useful in an emergency situation (when it is necessary to gather information in a short time), it is important to provide an opportunity for asking the patient to explain the answers to these questions in greater detail.
- **Leading questions** typically suggest the desired response, such as, "The infection seems to be getting better, don't you agree?" and thereby reduce the range of responses because the interviewee most commonly agrees with any leading statement. Highly emotional questions ("Where did you learn *that* injection technique?") also suggest the desired response and may be heard as challenging, provoking the interviewee to "attack" or become defensive, thereby blocking communication.
- **Probing** is a persistent questioning, a demand for more information than is given willingly. "Now tell me about . . ." This creates an uneasy feeling in the patient and may be interpreted as an invasion of privacy, resulting in a defensive response or withholding of information.
- **Agreeing/disagreeing** implies that the patient is "right" or "wrong" rather than promoting the patient's idea as separate from your own. This can block exploration of an issue. "I agree, that would be the thing to do" or "You didn't mean to do that, did you?"

---

attitude conveys competence, interest, kindness, thoroughness, orderliness, and confidence. It may be frightening for the patient if you convey the impression that you do not know what you are doing, or if you are awkward in performing tasks. Give the patient a clear explanation of the procedures you will be using. Then, proceed with the assessment according to the format you have previously chosen to gather and record the data: a nursing model (as suggested earlier), a systems approach (cardiovascular, respiratory, gastrointestinal, and so on), a head-to-toe approach (head, neck, chest, and so on), or a combination of these. The same format should be used each time you perform a physical assessment to lessen the possibility of omissions.

However, the patient's state of health/severity of condition may require that specific areas of the examination be done first. For example, when examining a patient with severe chest pain, you would probably choose to evaluate the pain and the cardiovascular system before addressing other areas of the body. The duration and length of any physical examination depends on circumstances, such as the condition of the patient and the urgency of the situation. You can offer emotional support and care where indicated. It is also important to provide the patient with as much feedback as possible and to take advantage of any teaching opportunities.

The nurse needs to exercise perceptual and observational skills during this aspect of information gathering.

Assessment Methods

To facilitate these observations, four methodologies have been developed using the senses of sight, hearing, touch, and smell:

1. *Inspection* is a systematic process of observation that is not limited to vision but also includes the senses of hearing and smell.

   Sight: Observing the skin for color, discolorations, lacerations; the lesion for drainage; the respiratory pattern for depth and symmetry; body language, movement and posture, use of extremities, presence of physical limitations; the face for expressions, and so on.

   Hearing: Listening to the nature of a cough; the integrity of a joint; the tone of a voice or content of interactions with others, and so on.

   Smell: Detecting significant odors.

2. *Palpation* is the touching or pressing of the external surface of the body with the fingers.

   Touch: Feeling a lump; noting temperature, degree of moistness.

   Pressure: Determining the character of a pulse, evaluating edema, or pinching to observe skin turgor.

   Probing deeper: Reveals muscle tone/tension or an abnormal pain response.

3. *Percussion* is the direct or indirect tapping of a specific body surface to ascertain information about underlying tissues or organs.

   Using fingertips: Tap the chest and listen for the sound indicating the presence or absence of fluid, masses, or consolidation.

   Using a percussion hammer: Tap the knee and observe the presence or absence of lower leg movement/reflexes.

4. *Auscultation* is listening for sounds within the body with the aid of a stethoscope and describing or interpreting them. This includes blood pressure as well as heart/fetal heart tones and lung, vascular, and bowel sounds.

Follow-up Considerations

Following the physical assessment, assist the patient as necessary. The patient may need to be helped down off the examining table for safety reasons or may require help with dressing.

Verification or clarification of communication associated with the physical assessment may also be needed. By repeating aloud what has been observed, the nurse gives the patient the opportunity to validate the accuracy of the information obtained and misunderstandings are avoided. For example,

Observation: "I noticed that you flinched when I palpated your abdomen"; *Response:* "Yes, your hand was cold and I'm ticklish."

LABORATORY AND DIAGNOSTIC STUDIES: SUPPORTING EVIDENCE

Laboratory and diagnostic studies are a part of the information-gathering stage. They aid in the management, maintenance, and restoration of health. Some tests are used to diagnose disease, while others are useful in following the course of a disease or adjusting therapy. Your knowledge about the purpose, procedure, and results of various scans, x-rays, performance tests (e.g., treadmill electrocardiogram, respiratory function), and numerous laboratory studies is necessary both for the success of the study and to promote timely nursing intervention and a positive patient outcome.

With laboratory tests, the origin of the test material does not always correlate to an organ or body system. For example, a urine test might be done to detect the presence of bilirubin and urobilinogen, which could indicate liver disease, biliary obstruction, or hemolytic disease. In some cases, the relationship of the test to the pathology is clear, while in others it is not. For example, obtaining renal function studies in the presence of cardiac failure. This is a result of the interrelationships between the various organs and systems of the body. In a few cases the results of a test are nonspecific, since they only indicate a disorder or abnormality and do not indicate where the cause of the problem is located. For example, an elevated sedimentation rate suggests the presence but not the location of an inflammatory process.

In evaluating laboratory tests, it is advisable to consider which drugs are being administered to the patient, since these may have the potential to blur or falsify results, creating a misleading diagnostic picture.

For example:
- Heparin will prolong blood clotting times.
- Oral iron preparations cause a false positive result when the stool is tested for occult blood.
- Pyridium can color the urine red.
- Use of promethazine can cause a false negative in a pregnancy test.

In some cases, it is necessary to note at what time the medication was administered, such as in determining drug levels or in determining the duration of the drug effect.

There are also several mechanisms that may alter the laboratory results through the introduction of interfering materials.

For example:
- Food that gives a yellow color to blood serum (e.g., carrots, yams) will alter a bilirubin test.
- Food may contribute to the presence of substances in body fluids, such as iodine, which may lead to a misdiagnosis of hypothyroidism.
- Intramuscular injections can elevate creatine phosphokinase (CPK) levels used to diagnose myocardial infarction.

ORGANIZING INFORMATION ELEMENTS

Clustering the Collected Data

Data gathered in the interview, in physical assessment, and from other records/sources are organized and recorded in a concise, systematic way and clustered into like categories. Various formats have been used to accomplish this, including a review of body systems. This body systems approach has been used by both medicine and nursing for many years but is actually more useful for the physician making a medical diagnosis than it is for the nurse identifying nursing diagnoses. Currently nursing is developing and fine-tuning its own tools for recording and clustering data. Organizing data using a nursing framework (Box 2–5) will assist you in focusing your attention and in choosing specific diagnostic labels to describe the data accurately. However, it is important to be aware of the advantages of each type of framework, and to follow the approach recommended by your school or hospital. Remember, consistency is the key. Work through Practice Activity 2–2 before continuing with the next section.

Reviewing and Validating Findings

VALIDATION is an ongoing process that occurs during the data collection phase and upon its completion, when the data are reviewed. The nurse reviews the data to be sure that what has been recorded is factual and to identify errors of omission or inconsistencies in the data that require additional investigation. As the nurse, you ask questions of the patient or others to verify your impressions; for example, "Tell me more about that" or "What I heard you say is . . ." Validating the information gathered can avoid the possibility of making wrong inferences or conclusions that can lead to incorrect goals and/or actions. This can be done by sharing your assumptions with the individuals involved and having them verify the accuracy of those conclusions.

Data that are grossly abnormal are rechecked, and objective and subjective data are compared for congruencies and/or inconsistencies. For example, the patient complains of right upper abdominal pain, although musculature appears relaxed and the patient does not flinch on abdominal palpation. Additional investigation reveals that the pain is episodic and usually follows meal times. Temporary factors that may affect the data are also identified/noted. For example, you note the patient's hands are very cold in comparison to the rest of her body. Upon questioning her, you discover she just washed her hands with cold water.

Finally, the patient may remember something, or feel more comfortable in sharing information with you, and although the data collected by any health-care professional are confidential, it may be appropriate or necessary to share the information. For example, you may have a greater opportunity to observe interactions between family members during the assessment process which could impact the diagnostic process and/or the plan of care. Some of these findings may need to be brought to the attention of other healthcare professionals, such as the physician, dietitian, or physical therapist. Sharing this additional data aids in collaborative planning of care.

VALIDATION—the process of assuring that data are factual.

BOX 2–5 ORGANIZING ASSESSMENT DATA USING A NURSING FRAMEWORK

The following data are representative of information you might have obtained for the patient database during your assessment of Martha. The data have been clustered in each of three nursing frameworks by means of the identifying numbers for each data element.

Assessment Data

1. 52-year-old female
2. High school teacher
3. Practicing Baptist
4. Divorced
5. One daughter in college
6. Fever 100°F (37.9°C)
7. Sharp severe pain, right upper quadrant radiating to right shoulder beginning 2 days ago
8. Hospitalized for kidney stones 4 years ago
9. Alert and oriented
10. Respirations 22, lungs clear, splinting with deep inspiration
11. Weight 148 lb (67.3 kg)
12. Three loose stools today, light tan color
13. Independent in self-care
14. Usually sleeps 6 to 8 hours each night
15. Takes pride in financial independence and being able to raise daughter without outside assistance
16. Menarche at age 13, menopause at age 45
17. Manages stress by prioritizing problems and dealing with smaller issues
18. Denies any allergies
19. Using liquid antacid without relief
20. Pulse 110, B/P 152/78 left arm/sitting

How you organize this data is dependent on the format you choose for recording. On occasion, data may be recorded in more than one section as the divisions/patterns are based on human responses instead of specific body systems. The above data could be recorded in three different nursing formats, thus:

DOENGES AND MOORHOUSE: DIAGNOSTIC DIVISIONS

Activity/Rest: 2, 9, 14
Circulation: 10, 20
Ego Integrity: 3, 4, 15, 17
Elimination: 8, 12
Food/Fluid: 11
Hygiene: 13
Neurosensory: 9

Pain/Comfort: 7, 19
Respiration: 10
Safety: 6, 18
Sexuality: 1, 5, 16
Social Interaction: 4, 5
Teaching/Learning: 8, 19

(Continued)

ORGANIZING DATA: DIAGNOSTIC DIVISIONS AND FUNCTIONAL HEALTH PATTERNS

Organize the data below according to diagnostic divisions and functional health patterns. *Place the number of the listed data next to the category where you believe it fits (see Table 2–1).*

1. 46-year-old male
2. Divorced, not currently involved in a relationship
3. Loan banker, laid off 7 months ago
4. Unsteady gait
5. Clothes rumpled, has not shaved for 2 days, dry skin
6. Eats two meals a day—donuts, sandwiches, meat and potatoes, no vegetables
7. Stools have been loose, 3 to 4 per day
8. Blood pressure 136/82, right arm/sitting, radial pulse 92
9. Alert and oriented
10. Catholic, not practicing
11. Sleeps usually 3 to 4 hours a night, awakens around 5:00 AM
12. "I've been drinking a lot lately." Bourbon 1 fifth per day
13. Worries about financial situation, unable to make support payments
14. Congested nonproductive cough
15. Complains of constant throbbing pain, left knee—old sports injury

Diagnostic Divisions

Activity/Rest: _____

Circulation: _____

Ego Integrity: _____

Elimination: _____

Food/Fluid: _____

Hygiene: _____

Neurosensory: _____

Pain/Comfort: _____

Respiration: _____

Safety: _____

Sexuality: _____

Social Interaction: _____

Teaching/Learning: _____

Functional Health Patterns:

Health Perception/Health Management: _____

Nutritional/Metabolic: _____

Elimination: _____

Activity/Exercise: _____

Cognitive/Perceptual: _____

Sleep/Rest: _____

Self-Perception/Self-Concept: _____

Role/Relationship: _____

Sexuality/Reproductive: _____

Coping/Stress Tolerance: _____

Value/Belief: _____

BOX 2-5 ORGANIZING ASSESSMENT DATA USING A NURSING FRAMEWORK (Continued)

GORDON: FUNCTIONAL HEALTH PATTERNS

Health Perception/Health Management: 7, 8, 19
Nutritional/Metabolic: 6, 10, 11, 18, 20
Elimination: 12
Activity/Exercise: 13, 10
Cognitive/Perceptual: 9
Sleep/Rest: 14

Self-Perception/Self-Concept: 15
Role/Relationship: 1, 2, 4, 5
Sexuality/Reproductive: 4, 5, 16
Coping/Stress Tolerance: 17
Value/Belief: 3

NANDA: HUMAN RESPONSE PATTERNS

Exchanging: 6, 8, 10, 11, 12, 18, 20
Communicating: 0
Relating: 1, 2, 4, 5, 16
Valuing: 3
Moving: 13, 14

Perceiving: 15
Knowing: 9
Feeling: 7, 19
Choosing: 17

SUMMARY

The assessment phase of the nursing process emphasizes and should provide a holistic view of the patient. The *generalized* assessment done during the overall gathering of data creates a profile of the patient. A *focused* assessment may be done to obtain more information about a specific issue that needs expansion or clarification. Both types of assessment are important, and complement each other. This allows the state of wellness of the patient, risk factors that may be present, and the patient's response to be clearly noted.

In the next step of the Nursing Process, the Diagnosis phase, diagnostic reasoning will be used to analyze/synthesize the information obtained from the patient database, identify the patient problems, and determine nursing diagnoses which form the basis for the development of the plan of care.

WORK PAGE: Chapter Two

1. Rewrite the following questions so that they are open-ended:

   a. You're feeling better after the respiratory treatment, aren't you?

   _____

   b. Have you taken your medicine today?

   _____

   c. Do you understand these directions?

   _____

2. Using the technique of reflection, write a question to clarify these patient responses:

   a. Do you think I should tell my doctor about my concern?

   _____

   b. What do you want to talk about today?

   _____

   c. I don't think I can go on without my husband.

   _____

   d. Do you think it is important to get married?

   _____

3. When might a closed-ended question be helpful? _____

4. Describe the three components of the patient database:

   _____

   _____

   _____

5. The four activities involved in the physical assessment are:

   _____

   _____

   _____

   _____

6. The patient database is important to the provision of patient care because _____

_____

7. For assessment purposes the difference between subjective data and objective data is _____

_____

8. Underline the subjective data, and circle the objective data in the following vignette:

> **Vignette:** Sally comes to the obstetric department for evaluation of her stage of labor. Back pains began about 3 hours ago during work as a respiratory therapist. Contractions are 5 minutes apart, lasting 40 seconds for the last 45 minutes. B/P 146/84, left arm/lying, pulse 110, respirations 24.
>
> Nauseated since a dinner of fried chicken 4 hours ago. Appears anxious and seems irritated that her physician is not here. Voided 1 hour ago, has not had a bowel movement for 2 days. Stopped smoking 8 months ago. Lungs clear. No allergies.
>
> Married, husband plans to attend the birth. Two children are in the care of their grandmother tonight. Appearance is well-groomed with a well-fitting maternity uniform and low-heeled shoes. Requests to leave contacts in to observe the birth. Last physical examination 1 week ago. Membranes have not ruptured. Due date is the middle of next week (2/25/92).

9. An important benefit for the nurse of doing "research" or reviewing available information before an

interview is _____

_____

10. An interview should be "requested" because _____

_____

11. Check those information resources that can be useful in helping the nurse to prepare for the interview:

_____ Family/significant other   _____ Physician notes

_____ Old medical records   _____ Textbooks/reference journals

_____ Diagnostic studies   _____ Other nurses/healthcare providers

12. Sensitivity of the nurse is important during the interview process to _____

_____

13. List three abilities of the nurse that are necessary in order to collect a relevant patient database.

(1) _____ (2) _____ (3) _____

14. Record and cluster the following data into the appropriate diagnostic divisions listed below. Refer to

Table 2 – 2 as needed for the type of data included in the specific divisions to assist you in clustering the data.

Vignette: Jennifer is a 3-year-old (1) female admitted to the outpatient surgery at 7:00 A.M. for (2) bilateral placement of tubes for chronic otitis media. (3) Has had nothing by mouth since midnight. (4) Uses diapers at night, (5) voided at 6:30 A.M. — clear yellow. She says, (6) "My ear hurts", as she pulls on her right ear. (7) Thick, grayish yellow drainage present in the right ear. (8) Appears scared, clutching mother tightly and trembling. (9) Rectal temperature 98°F (36.5°C), (10) BP 85/48 (left arm/lying), pulse 86/regular, (11) respirations 22/regular. (12) Skin warm, dry, color pink. (13) Right tympanic membrane dull, gray; perforation noted in central area. Mother reports, (14) "This is the second episode in two months." (15) Receiving Amoxicillin for the past week without improvement noted. In reviewing diagnostic studies, you note the (16) chest x-ray is clear and a (17) culture of the drainage reveals streptococcus pneumoniae.

DIAGNOSTIC DIVISIONS

Activity/rest: _____   Hygiene: _____   Safety: _____

Circulation: _____   Neurosensory: _____   Sexuality: _____

Ego integrity: _____   Pain/comfort: _____   Social interaction: _____

Elimination: _____   Respiration: _____   Teaching/learning: _____

Food/fluid: _____

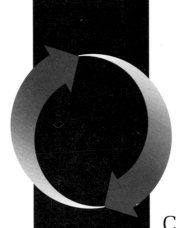

CHAPTER 3

The Diagnosis Phase: Problem Identification

ANA Standard 2: *Nursing diagnoses are derived from health status data.*

The second phase of the nursing process is often referred to as "**ANALYSIS**," as well as "**PROBLEM IDENTIFICATION**" or "**NURSING DIAGNOSIS**." Although all of these terms may be used interchangeably, the purpose of this step of the nursing process is to draw conclusions regarding a patient's specific problems or needs so that effective care can be planned and delivered. We have chosen to label this step of the nursing process "problem identification." To be more specific, problem identification is a process of data analysis using diagnostic reasoning (a form of clinical judgment) in which judgments, decisions, and conclusions are made about the *meaning* of the data collected, in order to determine whether or not nursing intervention is indicated.

The **DIAGNOSIS** of patient problems has been done by nurses on an informal basis since the early beginnings of the profession. The term came into

ANALYSIS—the process of examining and categorizing information to reach a conclusion about a patient's needs.

PROBLEM IDENTIFICATION—the second step of the Nursing Process, in which the data **33**

Table 3-1 NURSING DIAGNOSES (THROUGH 9TH NANDA CONFERENCE) 1990

Activity Intolerance
Activity Intolerance, high risk for
Adjustment, impaired
Airway Clearance, ineffective
Anxiety (specify level)
Aspiration, high risk for

Body Image Disturbance
Body Temperature, altered, high risk for
Bowel Incontinence
Breastfeeding, effective
Breastfeeding, ineffective
Breathing Pattern, ineffective

Cardiac Output, decreased
Communication, impaired verbal
Constipation
Constipation, colonic
Constipation, perceived
Coping, defensive
Coping, ineffective, individual

Decisional Conflict (specify)
Denial, ineffective
Diarrhea
Disuse Syndrome, high risk for
Diversional Activity Deficit
Dysreflexia

Family Coping, compromised
Family Coping, disabling
Family Coping, potential for growth
Family Processes, altered
Fatigue
Fear
Fluid Volume Deficit [active loss]
Fluid Volume Deficit [regulatory failure]
Fluid Volume Deficit, high risk for
Fluid Volume Excess

Gas Exchange, impaired
Grieving, anticipatory
Grieving, dysfunctional
Growth and Development, altered

Health Maintenance, altered
Health-Seeking Behaviors (specify)
Home Maintenance Management, impaired
Hopelessness
Hyperthermia
Hypothermia

Incontinence, functional
Incontinence, reflex
Incontinence, stress
Incontinence, total
Incontinence, urge
Infection, high risk for
Injury, high risk for

Knowledge Deficit [learning need] (specify)

Noncompliance [Compliance, altered] (specify)
Nutrition, altered, less than body requirements
Nutrition, altered, more than body requirements
Nutrition, altered, high risk for more than body requirements

Oral Mucous Membrane, altered

Pain [acute]
Pain, chronic
Parental Role Conflict
Parenting, altered
Parenting, altered, high risk for
Personal Identity Disturbance
Physical Mobility, impaired
Poisoning, high risk for
Posttrauma Response
Powerlessness
Protection, altered

Rape-Trauma Syndrome
Rape-Trauma Syndrome: compound reaction
Rape-Trauma Syndrome: silent reaction
Role Performance, altered

Self-Care Deficit: feeding, bathing/hygiene, dressing/grooming, toileting
Self-Esteem, chronic low
Self-Esteem, disturbance
Self-Esteem, situational low
Sensory-Perceptual Alterations (specify): visual, auditory, kinesthetic, gustatory, tactile, olfactory
Sexual Dysfunction
Sexuality Patterns, altered
Skin Integrity, impaired
Skin Integrity, impaired, high risk for
Sleep Pattern Disturbance
Social Interaction, impaired
Social Isolation
Spiritual Distress
Suffocation, high risk for
Swallowing Impaired

Thermoregulation, ineffective
Thought Processes, altered
Tissue Integrity, impaired
Tissue Perfusion, altered (specify): cerebral, cardiopulmonary, renal, gastrointestinal, peripheral
Trauma, high risk for

Unilateral Neglect
Urinary Elimination, altered patterns
Urinary Retention [acute/chronic]

Violence, high risk for, directed at self/others

NOTE: Information appearing in brackets [ ] has been added by the authors to clarify and facilitate the use of nursing diagnoses.

formal use by the nursing profession during the 1950s, although its meaning continued to be seen in the context of medical diagnosis. A group of interested nurses met and held a national conference in 1973. Their purpose was to identify the patient problems that fall within the scope of nursing, label them, and develop a classification system which could be used by nurses throughout the world. This group called these labels "nursing diagnoses." Regional workshops and conferences have since been held, and NANDA continues to meet every two years to review *their* work on the development of nursing diagnoses, as well as the work of other nursing groups representing various clinical specialties and healthcare settings.

ANA standards of practice were developed in 1973, and with the acceptance of the *ANA Social Policy Statement* in 1980, which defined nursing as the "diagnosis and treatment of human responses to actual and potential health problems," the movement for broad use of a common language was enhanced. The system developed by NANDA reflects a standard terminology which is accepted by ANA and various specialty groups and which is being used across the United States and in many countries around the world. The NANDA list has also been proposed for inclusion in the World Health Organization's tenth edition of *International Classification of Diseases* (ICD-10).

Today, the use of the nursing process and nursing diagnoses is rapidly becoming an integral part of an effective system of nursing practice. It is a system which can be used within existing conceptual frameworks, because it is a generic approach adaptable to all academic and clinical settings.

DEFINING NURSING DIAGNOSIS

The term *nursing diagnosis* has been used as both a verb and a noun. This may result in confusion. *Nursing diagnosis* is used as a noun in reference to the work of NANDA. For the purposes of this text, nursing diagnosis will refer to the NANDA list of nursing diagnosis labels (Table 3–1) that form the stem of the **PATIENT DIAGNOSTIC STATEMENT.**

Although nurses work within the nursing, medical, and psychosocial domains, nursing's phenomena of concern are patterns of human response, not disease processes. Therefore, nursing diagnoses do not parallel medical/psychiatric diagnoses but do involve independent nursing activities as well as collaborative roles and actions.

The nursing diagnosis is a conclusion drawn from the data collected about a patient which serves as a means of describing a health problem amenable to treatment by nurses. A uniform or standardized way of identifying, focusing on, and labeling specific phenomena allows the nurse to deal effectively with individual patient responses.

Although there are differing definitions of the term *nursing diagnosis*, NANDA has accepted the following working definition:

> Nursing diagnosis is a clinical judgment about individual, family, or community responses to actual and potential health problems/life processes. Nursing diagnoses provide the basis for selection of nursing interventions to achieve outcomes for which the nurse is accountable.

The nursing diagnosis is as correct as the present data will allow because it is supported by the immediate data collected. It says what the patient's

collected are analyzed and, through the process of diagnostic reasoning, specific patient diagnostic statements are created.

NURSING DIAGNOSIS —*Noun:* a label approved by NANDA identifying specific patient problems/ needs. The means of describing health problems amenable to treatment by nurses; may be physical, sociologic, or psychologic. *Verb:* the process of identifying specific patient problems/needs; used by some as the title of the second step of the nursing process.

DIAGNOSIS— identification of a disease/condition or human response by a scientific evaluation of signs/symptoms, history, and diagnostic studies.

PATIENT DIAGNOSTIC STATEMENT—the outcome of the diagnostic reasoning process; a three-part statement identifying the patient's problem/need, the etiology of the problem/need, and the associated signs/symptoms.

Distinguishing between Medical and Nursing Diagnoses . . .

- *Medical Diagnoses* are illnesses/conditions such as diabetes, heart failure, hepatitis, cancer, and pneumonia. The medical diagnosis usually does *not* change.

- *Nursing Diagnoses* address human responses to actual and potential illnesses/conditions such as Activity Intolerance; Health Maintenance, altered; Airway Clearance, ineffective; Self-Care Deficit. The nursing diagnosis may change as the patient's problem progresses toward resolution.

SIGN—objective or observable evidence or manifestation of a health problem.

SYMPTOM— subjectively perceptible change in the body or its functions that indicates disease or the kind or phases of disease.

situation is at the *present* time and reflects changes in the patient's condition as they occur. Each decision the nurse makes is time-dependent and, with additional information gathered at a later point in time, these decisions may change. Unlike medical diagnoses, nursing diagnoses change as the patient progresses through various stages of illness/maladaptation, to resolution of the problem or to the conclusion of the condition. For example, for a patient undergoing cardiac surgery, initial problems/needs may be Pain, Cardiac Output, Airway Clearance, and High Risk for Infection. As the patient progresses, problems/needs may shift to Activity Intolerance, Knowledge Deficit, and Role Performance.

THE USE OF NURSING DIAGNOSIS

Although not yet comprehensive, the current NANDA list of diagnostic labels defines/refines professional nursing activity. The list of labels is now at a point where nurses need to use the proposed diagnoses on a daily basis, becoming familiar with the parameters of each individual diagnosis, and identifying its strengths and weaknesses, thus promoting research and further development.

The question is frequently asked: "Why should we use nursing diagnosis . . . what is its value to the nursing profession?" There are many benefits which the use of nursing diagnoses can provide. The accurate choice of a nursing diagnosis to label a patient problem/need:

- *Gives Nurses a Common Language:* Promotes improved communication among nurses, between shifts and units, other healthcare providers and alternate care settings.

  For example: Using the nursing diagnosis "Airway Clearance, ineffective" instead of "Difficulty breathing" conveys a distinct image. When hearing the former, a clear picture begins to develop in your mind, as your thoughts focus on the musculature of the upper airway, mucus production, and cough effort. With the second label, you do not have a clear idea as to what is happening with this patient, and you question whether the patient is experiencing a problem of maintaining an airway, movement of the chest, or perfusion to the lungs.

  This improved communication may result in improved quality and continuity of the care provided to the patient.

- *Promotes Identification of Appropriate Goals:* Aids in the choice of correct nursing interventions to alleviate the identified problem/need, and provides guidance for evaluation. Whereas nursing actions were once based on variables such as **SIGNS** and **SYMPTOMS**, test results, and a medical diagnosis, nursing diagnosis is a uniform way of identifying, focusing on, and dealing with specific patient responses to actual and potential health problems/needs (i.e., the phenomena of concern for nurses).

  For example: "High Risk for Infection" versus "Presence of Urinary Catheter." The high risk or potential threat of an infection brings to mind specific goals/outcomes and interventions to protect this patient, but what is your concern, if any, with the urinary catheter?

- *Provides Acuity Information:* Ranks the amount of work activity which nursing care of a given patient requires. Can serve as a basis for patient classification systems. This method of ranking can be used to determine individual staffing needs. It can also serve as documentation which provides justification for third-party reimbursement.

  For example: Nursing diagnoses can be given different, weighted values according to the degree of nursing involvement required; that is, "Gas Exchange, impaired," may require a considerable amount of skilled nursing time in order to promote adequate ventilation, to provide oxygen and respiratory treatments, and to monitor laboratory studies. "Acute Urinary Retention" may require a shorter period of time to insert a catheter into the bladder and periodically measure the urine output.

  In addition, some third-party payers (such as medicare and other insurance companies) include nursing diagnoses when considering extended length of stay or delayed discharge.

- *Can Create a Standard for Nursing Practice:* Provides a foundation for quality improvement programs, a means of evaluating nursing practice, and a mechanism of costing-out delivery of nursing care.

  For example: Did the nursing interventions address and resolve the problem? Did the patient experience the desired result (for instance, alleviation of pain)? Were the goals met, or is there documentation of the reasons why they were not met? Were the expected outcomes changed to meet changing patient needs?

- *Provides a Quality Improvement Base:* Clinicians, administrators, educators, and researchers can document, validate, and/or alter the process of care delivery, which then improves the profession.

  For example: The use of universally understood labels enhances retrieval of specific data for review to determine accuracy; to validate and/or change nursing actions related to specific nursing diagnoses; and also to evaluate an individual nurse's performance.

> Remember . . .
> nursing diagnoses may be a *physical, sociologic,* or *psychologic* finding:
>
> **Physical Nursing Diagnoses**
> include those which pertain to circulation (for example, Tissue Perfusion), ventilation (for example, Airway Clearance), elimination (for example, Constipation), and so on.
>
> **Psychosocial Nursing Diagnoses**
> include those that pertain to the mind (for example, Thought Processes), emotion (for example, Anxiety), or lifestyle/ relationships (for example, Sexuality Patterns, altered, or Social Isolation).

IDENTIFYING PATIENT PROBLEMS/NEEDS

During the Assessment phase, the collection, clustering, and validation of patient data flows directly into the Problem Identification phase of the nursing process, as the nurse begins to *sense* problems.

Diagnostic Reasoning: Analyzing the Patient Database

Identifying patient problems/needs and then selecting a nursing diagnosis label involves the use of experience, expertise, and intuition on the part of the nurse. There are six steps involved in this problem identification process.

BOX 3–1 NURSING DIAGNOSES ORGANIZED ACCORDING TO DIAGNOSTIC DIVISIONS

After data have been collected and areas of concern/need have been identified, the nurse is directed to the Diagnostic Divisions framework to review the list of nursing diagnoses that fall within the individual categories. This will assist with the choice of the specific diagnostic labels to accurately describe the data from the patient database. Then, with the addition of etiology (when known) and signs and symptoms, the patient diagnostic statement emerges.

Diagnostic Division: Activity/Rest

Ability to engage in necessary/desired activities of life (work and leisure) and to obtain sleep/rest

DIAGNOSES

Activity Intolerance
Activity Intolerance, high risk
Disuse Syndrome, high risk for
Diversional Activity Deficit
Fatigue
Sleep Pattern Disturbance

Diagnostic Division: Circulation

Ability to transport oxygen and nutrients necessary to meet cellular needs

DIAGNOSES

Cardiac Output, decreased
Dysreflexia
Tissue Perfusion, altered (specify): cerebral, cardiopulmonary, renal, gastrointestinal, peripheral

Diagnostic Division: Ego Integrity

Ability to develop and use skills and behaviors to integrate and manage life experiences

DIAGNOSES

Adjustment, impaired
Anxiety (specify level)
Body Image Disturbance
Coping, defensive
Coping, ineffective, individual
Decisional Conflict (specify)
Denial, ineffective
Fear
Grieving, anticipatory
Grieving, dysfunctional
Hopelessness
Personal Identity Disturbance
Posttrauma Response
Powerlessness

(Continued)

BOX 3–1 NURSING DIAGNOSES ORGANIZED ACCORDING TO DIAGNOSTIC DIVISIONS (Continued)

Rape-Trauma Syndrome
Rape-Trauma Syndrome: compound reaction   Rape-Trauma Syndrome: silent reaction
Self-Esteem, chronic low
Self-Esteem Disturbance
Self-Esteem, situational low
Spiritual Distress

Diagnostic Division: Elimination

Ability to excrete waste products
DIAGNOSES

Bowel Incontinence
Constipation
Constipation, colonic
Constipation, perceived
Diarrhea
Incontinence, functional
Incontinence, reflex
Incontinence, stress
Incontinence, total
Incontinence, urge
Urinary Elimination, altered patterns
Urinary Retention [acute/chronic]

Diagnostic Divisions: Food/Fluid

Ability to maintain intake of and use nutrients and liquids to meet physiologic needs
DIAGNOSES

Breastfeeding, effective
Breastfeeding, ineffective
Fluid Volume Deficit [Active loss]
Fluid Volume Deficit [Regulatory failure]
Fluid Volume Deficit, high risk for
Fluid Volume Excess
Nutrition, altered, less than body requirements
Nutrition, altered, more than body requirements
Nutrition, altered, high risk for more than body requirements
Oral Mucous Membrane, altered
Swallowing, impaired

Diagnostic Division: Hygiene

Ability to perform activities of daily living
DIAGNOSES

Self-Care Deficit: feeding, bathing/hygiene, dressing/grooming, toileting

(Continued)

BOX 3–1 NURSING DIAGNOSES ORGANIZED ACCORDING TO DIAGNOSTIC DIVISIONS (Continued)

Diagnostic Division: Neurosensory

Ability to perceive, integrate, and respond to internal and external cues
  DIAGNOSES

> Sensory-Perceptual Alterations (specify): visual, auditory, kinesthetic, gustatory, tactile, olfactory
> Thought Processes, altered
> Unilateral Neglect

Diagnostic Division: Pain/Comfort

Ability to control internal/external environment to maintain comfort
  DIAGNOSES

> Pain [acute]
> Pain, chronic

Diagnostic Division: Respiration

Ability to provide and use oxygen to meet physiologic needs
  DIAGNOSES

> Airway Clearance, ineffective
> Aspiration, high risk for
> Breathing Pattern, ineffective
> Gas Exchange, impaired

Diagnostic Division: Safety

Ability to provide safe, growth promoting environment
  DIAGNOSES

> Body Temperature, altered, high risk for
> Health Maintenance, altered
> Home Maintenance Management, impaired
> Hyperthermia
> Hypothermia
> Infection, high risk for
> Injury, high risk for
> Physical Mobility, impaired
> Poisoning, high risk for
> Protection, altered
> Skin Integrity, impaired
> Skin Integrity, impaired, high risk for
> Suffocation, high risk for
> Thermoregulation, ineffective
> Tissue Integrity, impaired
> Trauma, high risk for
> Violence, high risk for, directed at self/others

(Continued)

BOX 3-1 NURSING DIAGNOSES ORGANIZED ACCORDING TO DIAGNOSTIC DIVISIONS (*Continued*)

Diagnostic Division: Sexuality

[Component of Ego Integrity and Social Interaction] Ability to meet requirements/characteristics of male/female role

DIAGNOSES

> Sexual Dysfunction
> Sexuality Patterns, altered

Diagnostic Division: Social Interaction

Ability to establish and maintain relationships

DIAGNOSES

> Communication, impaired verbal
> Family Coping, compromised
> Family Coping, disabling
> Family Coping, potential for growth
> Family Processes, altered
> Parental Role conflict
> Parenting, altered
> Parenting, altered, high risk for
> Role Performance, altered
> Social Interaction, impaired
> Social Isolation

Diagnostic Division: Teaching/Learning

Ability to incorporate and use information to achieve healthy lifestyle/ optimal wellness

DIAGNOSES

> Growth and Development, altered
> Health-Seeking Behaviors (specify)
> Knowledge Deficit [learning need] (specify)
> Noncompliance [Compliance, altered] (specify)

These steps comprise the activities of diagnostic reasoning and result in the creation of a patient diagnostic statement which identifies the patient problem, suggests its potential cause or etiology, and notes its signs and symptoms. This is known as the (P)roblem, (E)tiology, and (S)igns and symptoms (or P E S format).

STEP ONE: PROBLEM-SENSING

Data are reviewed and analyzed to identify **CUES** (signs and symptoms) suggesting patient problems or needs that can be described by nursing diagnosis labels. If the data have been recorded in a nursing format (e.g., Diagnostic Divisions, Functional Health Patterns, or Human Responses), the nurse is automatically guided to specific groups of nursing diagnoses when certain

CUE—a signal that indicates a possible need/direction for care.

cues from the data are identified (see Box 3–1). This helps to focus your attention on appropriate diagnoses. Reviewing the NANDA definitions of specific diagnoses (Appendix A) can be of further assistance in deciding between two or more similar diagnostic labels; for instance, there are five different diagnoses for urinary incontinence (see Step 4, below).

> **For example:** When using the Diagnostic Divisions format, body temperature is recorded in the Safety section. When the patient manifests an elevation of temperature, the nurse would review the diagnostic labels under Safety to find a possible fit, such as *Hyperthermia* or *Infection, high risk for.* At the same time, cues are noted in other sections of the database which may be combined with fever or be totally unrelated. In fact, cues may have relevance in more than one section, as you can see in Box 3–2.

STEP TWO: RULE-OUT PROCESS

Alternative explanations are considered for the identified cues to determine which nursing diagnosis label may be most appropriate. This step is crucial to the establishment of an adequate list of diagnostic statements. As you compare and contrast the relationships among and between data, etiologic factors are identified within or between categories based on an understanding of the biologic, physical, and behavioral sciences.

> **For example:** Although *Hyperthermia* or *Infection, high risk for,* were suggested during the first step of diagnostic reasoning, another consideration might be *Fluid Volume Deficit.* In another example, cues of increased tension, restlessness, elevated pulse rate, and reported apprehension may initially be thought to indicate *Anxiety.* However, a similar diagnosis of *Fear* should be considered, as well as the possibility that these cues may be physiologically based, needing medical treatment and nursing interventions related to learning needs/monitoring.

If you encounter difficulty in choosing a nursing diagnosis label, the questions in Box 3–3 may provide additional guidance.

STEP THREE: SYNTHESIZING THE DATA

SYNTHESIZING— viewing all data as a whole to provide a comprehensive picture of the patient.

Looking at all the data as a whole (including information collected by other members of the healthcare team) can provide a comprehensive picture of the patient in relation to the past, present, and future health status. This is called **SYNTHESIZING** the data. The suggested nursing diagnosis label is combined with the identified related factor(s) and cues to create a hypothesis, for example, the nursing diagnosis label *Fluid Volume Deficit;* related factor, hemorrhage; cues, dark urine, dry mouth/lips, low blood pressure, fever.

STEP FOUR: EVALUATING OR CONFIRMING THE HYPOTHESIS

ETIOLOGY— identified causes and/or contributing factors

Test the hypothesis for appropriate fit; that is, you review the NANDA nursing diagnosis and definition. Then, compare the suggested **ETIOLOGY** with

BOX 3-2   WALKING THROUGH THE USE OF DIAGNOSTIC DIVISIONS

During the Assessment phase, the following data were obtained from Robert.

Respiration

Subjective

Dyspnea (related to): activity—climbing stairs, walking two blocks

Cough/sputum: hacking cough with moderate amount of thick greenish mucus past 6 days

History of Bronchitis: chronic   **Asthma:** no

           Tuberculosis: no   **Emphysema:** no

           Recurrent pneumonia: second episode in 6 months

           Exposure to noxious fumes: no

Smokes: filters   **Pk/day:** ½ pkg   **# of pack years:** 30

Use of respiratory aids: inhaler & PO meds   **Oxygen:** 2.5 L/cannula

Objective

Respiratory: Rate: 32   **Depth:** shallow   **Symmetry:** equal

Use of accessory muscles: intercostals and leaning forward

    Nasal flaring: no

Fremitus: decreased   **Egophony:** normal   **Percussion:** hyper-resonant

Breath sounds: diminished, basalar crackles bilateral, scattered rhonchi, limited, clearing with cough

Cyanosis: mucous membranes—pale   **Clubbing of fingers:** slight

Sputum characteristics: as above

Mentation/restlessness: alert

Other: verbal responses slow; breathless

Having reviewed the collected data for this patient with pneumonia and noting cues (signs and symptoms) in the Respiration section of the database, you are referred to the Respiration section of the Diagnostic Divisions. Four possible labels are suggested: Airway Clearance, ineffective; Aspiration, high risk for; Breathing pattern, ineffective; and Gas Exchange, impaired.

    In addition, the complaint of dyspnea with activity would refer you to the Activity/Rest section of the Diagnostic Divisions, where the effects of this condition on both activity and sleep would also be considered: Activity Intolerance; Activity Intolerance, high risk for; Disuse Syndrome, high risk for; Diversional Activity deficit; Fatigue; and Sleep Pattern disturbance.

BOX 3–3 QUESTIONS TO ASK YOURSELF WHEN THE NURSING DIAGNOSIS LABEL IS UNCLEAR

When the nursing diagnosis label is unclear, the nurse can ask these questions:

1. What are my concerns about this patient?
2. Can I/am I doing something about it?
3. Can the overall risk be reduced by nursing intervention?

For example, in the pediatric patient, fever is often a major concern. Questions to ask might be:

- *What are the concerns about the fever?*—The patient may convulse.
- *Can I do something about it?*—Try to bring the temperature down and make the environment safe.
- *Can the overall risk be reduced by nursing interventions?*—Yes, the risk of convulsions can be reduced if the temperature is lowered; or if convulsions do occur, measures can be taken to protect the patient from injury.

Conclusion: The Nursing Diagnosis would be *High Risk for Injury;* and the patient diagnostic statement would be *High Risk for Injury: seizures related to prolonged high fever.*

BOX 3–4 ELEMENTS OF NANDA NURSING DIAGNOSIS LABELS

Appendix A supplies a complete listing of NANDA Nursing Diagnosis labels, which will be helpful to you as you work through the exercises in this chapter and throughout the book. Take a moment to identify the key elements of the diagnostic label, "Fluid Volume Deficit," and then turn to Appendix A and try to locate the diagnosis in the listing. It is important to become familiar with the listing, so that you can find information quickly in the clinical setting.

Fluid Volume Deficit

- *Definition:* The state in which an individual experiences vascular, cellular, or intracellular dehydration
- *Related Factors:* Active loss
- *Defining Characteristics:* Decreased urine output, output greater than intake, concentrated urine, sudden weight loss, decreased venous filling, hemoconcentration, increased serum sodium, thirst, hypotension, decreased skin turgor, increased pulse rate, dry skin/mucous membranes, increased body temperature, weakness, decreased pulse volume/pressure, change in mental state.

NANDA's **RELATED FACTORS** or **RISK FACTORS** and compare the identified cues with NANDA's Defining Characteristics, paying special attention to critical or major characteristics which should be present for the diagnosis to be confirmed. This reduces the possibility of making a diagnostic error. Take a moment to look at Box 3–4. As you can see by reviewing the NANDA diagnostic label, Fluid Volume Deficit (in Box 3–4), related factors (etiology) include active loss with defining characteristics (signs/symptoms) such as concentrated urine, dry mucous membranes, hypotension, and increased body temperature. In addition, another defining characteristic is hemoconcentration, which you noted when you reviewed the patient's CBC.

STEP FIVE: LIST THE PATIENT'S PROBLEMS/NEEDS

Based on the data obtained from Steps 3 and 4, the nursing diagnosis label is combined with the etiology and signs/symptoms, if present, to finalize the *patient diagnostic statement*, for example, Fluid Volume Deficit related to hemorrhage as evidenced by dark urine, dry mucous membranes, fever, hypotension, and hemoconcentration. This individualized diagnosis reflects the P E S format for a three-part diagnostic statement, as described in Box 3–5. A diagnostic statement will be needed for <u>each</u> problem/need you identify.

STEP SIX: REEVALUATE THE PROBLEM LIST

Be sure all areas of concern are noted. Once all nursing diagnoses are identified, list them according to priority and classify them according to status: an active problem/need; a potential or high risk problem/need; or a resolved problem/need. Box 3–6 explains this status classification.

- *Active Diagnoses*—have already occurred and require some form of current action or intervention.

   For example: Ruth is admitted for a medical workup for problems with bladder function related to her diagnosis of multiple sclerosis. An active problem might be *Urinary Retention*.

- *High Risk or Potential Diagnoses*—may occur/recur, especially if intervention of some kind is not done to prevent them.

   For example: Ruth's multiple sclerosis has been in remission, but she has had difficulty in the past with physical mobility. This past problem must be considered when planning this patient's care in order to minimize the possibility of recurrence. A potential problem would then be identified as *Physical Mobility, impaired, risk for*.

- *Resolved Diagnoses*—are those that no longer need action.

   For example: Ruth once suffered a decubitus ulcer (Skin Integrity, impaired), but she has learned techniques to prevent recurrence of this problem, and her skin is in good condition. Therefore, as long as Ruth is able to participate in or direct her own care, this is of no significant concern to you at this time.

Finally, validate the diagnostic conclusions/impressions with a colleague and/or the patient. This helps to reduce the possibility of **DIAGNOSTIC ERRORS** and/or omissions as discussed in Box 3–7. Inclusion of the patient/significant

---

responsible for the presence of a specific patient problem/need.

RELATED FACTOR— the condition or situation which appears to demonstrate some type of patterned relationship with a specific nursing diagnosis; forms the *related to* component of the patient diagnostic statement.

RISK FACTOR—the condition or situation that may lead to the development/ recurrence of a patient problem/specific nursing diagnosis.

Examples of Active Problems:

   Skin Integrity, impaired
   Pain [acute]
   Self-Care Deficit
   Knowledge Deficit [treatment needs]

Examples of High Risk Problems:

   Infection, high risk for
   Adjustment, impaired
   Body Image Disturbance

DIAGNOSTIC ERROR —a mistaken assumption leading to a wrong conclusion.

BOX 3-5 COMPONENTS OF THE PATIENT DIAGNOSTIC STATEMENT: PROBLEM, ETIOLOGY, AND SIGNS AND SYMPTOMS (P E S)

P = *Problem/Need* is the name or diagnostic label which is identified from the NANDA list. The key to accurate nursing diagnosis is problem identification which focuses attention on a current, high risk or potential physical or behavioral response that interferes with the quality of life the patient is used to or desires. It deals with concerns, of the patient/significant other(s) and the nurse, which require nursing intervention and management.

E = *Etiology* is the suspected cause of/or reason for the response which has been identified from the assessment (patient database). The nurse makes inferences based on knowledge and expertise, such as understanding of pathophysiology, and situational or developmental factors. The etiology is stated as "related to." Note: One problem may have several suspected causes, such as Self-esteem disturbance, related to lack of positive feedback and dysfunctional family system.

S = *Signs and Symptoms* are the manifestations (or cues) identified in the assessment which substantiate the nursing diagnosis. They are stated as "evidenced by" followed by a list of subjective and objective data. It is important to note that High Risk or potential diagnoses are *not* accompanied by signs and symptoms because the problem has not yet actually occurred. In this instance, the "S" component of the problem statement is omitted and the "E" component would be replaced by an itemization of the identified risk factors which suggest that the diagnosis could occur. For example: Infection, high risk for, related to malnutrition, and invasive procedures.

BOX 3-6 STATUS CLASSIFICATION OF PATIENT PROBLEMS/NEEDS

- *Active:* A problem/need that is currently present and manifested by signs and symptoms. In recording the problem/need, you use a three-part P E S statement. *Altered Urinary Patterns related to neuromuscular impairment evidenced by dribbling, 250 cc residual urine.*
- *High Risk or Potential:* A problem/need that you believe could develop, but since it has not yet occurred, there are no signs or symptoms, only "risk factors." The problem/need would be written as a two-part statement. *Impaired Physical Mobility, high risk for, related to neuromuscular impairment.*
- *Resolved:* A problem/need which no longer requires intervention. Since the problem no longer exists, no diagnostic statement is needed.

other(s) promotes understanding and participation in the planning of individualized care.

Other Considerations for Problem Identification

The medical/psychiatric diagnosis can provide a starting point for identifying associated patient problems (problem-sensing). While they can suggest
several nursing diagnoses, these nursing diagnoses must be supported by cues
in the patient database.

> **For example:** In the presence of a myocardial infarction, the patient
> often suffers pain, anxiety, and activity intolerance and requires
> teaching activities. In addition, the patient may be at high risk for
> alteration of cardiac output, tissue perfusion, and fluid volume excess.
> These problems and needs are not necessarily present in each patient
> with this condition. One patient may actually be pain-free, while
> another patient could demonstrate a sleep disturbance or report
> spiritual distress. Therefore a medical diagnosis can be an initial point
> for problem-sensing, but the validity of a nursing diagnosis depends
> upon the presence of individually appropriate supporting data.

The patient's or family member's understanding of normal body function,
individual expectations, or mistaken perceptions may result in the belief that
a problem exists, even in the absence of diagnostically appropriate supporting
data. Even though the problem seems to exist *only* in the mind of the patient/
significant other, it needs to be addressed and resolved in order to promote
optimal wellness.

> **For example:**
>
> 1. The parent of a child with cancer may believe that the child is
>   incapable of self-care activities even though the child's level of
>   function and development would indicate otherwise. This then is
>   not a patient problem with self-care but rather the parent's
>   problem—possibly, Family Coping, ineffective: compromised.
> 2. A female patient may believe that sexual desire normally disap-
>   pears after menopause/hysterectomy, and the fact that it has not
>   indicates to her that something is wrong. Although sexual dys-
>   function may have occurred, the assessment reveals inadequate
>   information and misconceptions. Therefore, the nursing diag-
>   nosis is Knowledge Deficit: normal sexual functioning.
> 3. An elderly, confused patient, with a diagnosis of Alzheimer's
>   disease, is found wandering in the day room. She has soiled
>   herself and is smearing feces on the walls and couch. The prob-
>   lem would not be one of bowel elimination but of Thought
>   Processes, impaired. Interventions would be addressed to the
>   solution of behavioral management rather than only to a bowel
>   control program.

As noted in the above examples, it is important to "reduce" the problem
to its basic component in order to focus interventions on the "roots" of the

---

BOX 3-7 POTENTIAL ERRORS IN CHOOSING A NURSING DIAGNOSIS

- **Overlooking Cues** resulting in a missed diagnosis can lead to worsening of the problem.

    For example: A patient complains of discomfort at the insertion site of an intravenous catheter (IV). You notice the area is slightly reddened but fail to consider the *high risk for infection*. As a result, the patient develops sepsis or a blood infection requiring emergency intervention.

- **Making a Diagnosis with an Insufficient Database** can lead in the wrong direction, wasting valuable time and resources.

    For example: The patient displays signs of anxiety. Without additional assessment, you administer a tranquilizer on the belief that the signs and symptoms are psychologically based. Later, when checking the patient, you find signs of cyanosis, suggesting inadequate oxygenation. Thus, the anxiety probably was at least in part physiologically based and needed other nursing interventions.

- **Stereotyping** leads to treating all patients in the same way and negates individualization.

    For example: In a medical-surgical setting, the assumption is often made that a patient with a psychiatric diagnosis is apt to become violent.

---

human response. This simplifies care and increases the likelihood of a timely and satisfactory resolution.

As a beginner, it is advisable to use the NANDA list in Appendix A when choosing a diagnostic label. However, as the list is still in a state of evolution, "holes" may exist. With practice and experience, the nurse may very well have occasion to identify a problem/need that is treatable with nursing interventions but for which there is no appropriate NANDA label. In this situation, the diagnosis should be stated clearly using the P E S format and then reviewed with other nursing colleagues to verify that the meaning and intent are accurately communicated. Finally, the work should be documented and submitted to NANDA for consideration.

INTUITION—*a sense of something that is not clearly evidenced by known facts.*

Experienced nurses may use **INTUITION** to arrive at a conclusion as an integral part of the diagnostic reasoning process. This use of intuition needs to be encouraged. Paying attention to the feelings or sense of something for which there is no visible data can add an important dimension to the diagnostic reasoning process. While checking, rechecking, and validating these impressions are crucial to the appropriate use of intuition (in order to avoid errors in judgment), the responsibly applied use of intuition can lead to insights not available in any other way.

Finally, the process of problem identification may be assisted by entering the patient database into a computer. The software program may offer you a list of nursing diagnoses which frequently occur correlated to specific medical diagnoses, or it may suggest possible nursing diagnoses based on cues that the program identifies. Such online diagnostic software is a support tool and does not eliminate the nurse's need to use the diagnostic reasoning process to identify and formulate appropriate patient diagnostic statements *independently* of the computer recommendations.

WRITING A PATIENT DIAGNOSTIC STATEMENT: USING P E S

As NANDA's list of nursing diagnosis labels increases, and issues of **WELLNESS** are addressed, the focus of a nursing diagnosis may not be limited solely to problems but may also include the patient's needs and strengths as well. For this reason, we have chosen to identify the *outcome* of the diagnostic reasoning process as the Patient Diagnostic Statement instead of the commonly used term "Patient Problem."

Using the **P E S FORMAT** as previously outlined, the problem/need, etiology, and signs and symptoms (or risk factors) are combined into a "neutral" statement avoiding value-laden or judgmental language. The use of ambiguous or judgmental terms such as "too often," "uncooperative," or "manipulative" can lead to misunderstandings on the part of the reader. Patients may become defensive, other readers may be influenced to make an inaccurate or biased decision, and the outcome of treatment may be negatively influenced.

The *problem* and *etiology* sections of the diagnostic statement are joined by the phrase "related to." Phrases such as "due to" or "caused by" indicate a specific causal link which may not exist, and should therefore be avoided. "Related to" suggests a connection between the nursing diagnosis and the identified factors, leaving open the possibility that there may be other contributing factors not yet recognized.

When writing a diagnostic statement, remember to include qualifiers or quantifiers as indicated in the NANDA list (e.g., Anxiety, severe . . .). If the term "specify" is noted with a diagnostic label, it is important that the correct information be provided to make the communication clear.

> **For example:** Tissue Perfusion, altered: <u>cerebral</u>; or Knowledge Deficit: <u>care of the newborn</u>.

By definition, nursing diagnoses identify patient problems/needs that can be positively impacted, or possibly prevented, by nursing actions. Some diagnoses permit a greater degree of independent function, while others are more collaborative in nature. This may be visualized as a continuum without a fixed midpoint differentiating independent from dependent actions (Fig. 3–1). Furthermore, the extent of independent function is influenced by the individual nurse's experience, level of expertise, work setting, and presence of established **PROTOCOLS** or Standards of Care. For this reason, the authors recommend that nurses identify the nursing component and appropriate interventions for any patient problem, instead of labeling independent versus **COLLABORATIVE PROBLEMS** or potential complications.

> **For example:**
> • In the patient who is hemorrhaging, the nursing component

WELLNESS—a state of optimal health, physical and psychosocial.

P E S—format for combining a patient problem label, etiology, and signs/symptoms to create an individualized diagnostic statement.

PROTOCOL—written guidelines of steps to be taken for providing patient care in a particular situation/condition.

COLLABORATIVE PROBLEM—a need identified by another discipline that will contain a nursing component requiring nursing intervention and/or monitoring.

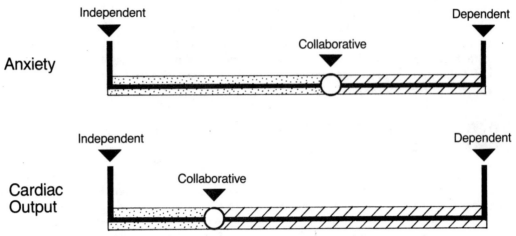

Figure 3-1 Representative comparison of degree of independent nursing function in two nursing diagnoses. Nursing diagnoses have a varying degree of independent function, and nursing actions can be identified for any patient situation. As shown in this diagram, the nursing diagnosis "Anxiety" has a high degree of independent nursing actions, while "Cardiac Output" has a lower degree.

would be <u>Fluid Volume Deficit</u> and the nurse would not only monitor the problem, but would provide assurance to the patient, and take action to control the blood loss.
- The presence of a subclavian IV catheter has concerns of <u>High Risk for Infection</u>, with implications for sterile dressing changes and observation of the site.
- A low serum potassium level may result in dysrhythmias that can be addressed in <u>Cardiac Output, altered high risk for</u>, requiring ECG interpretation, possible limiting of activities, provision of potassium-containing foods/fluids as appropriate, and other interventions based on protocols.

Box 3-8 summarizes some common errors in creating and writing the patient diagnostic statement. Box 3-9 demonstrates how possible nursing diagnoses can be linked or associated with medical disorders, to allow the nurse rapid identification of nursing diagnoses for a particular patient situation.

BOX 3–8 COMMON ERRORS IN CREATING AND WRITING THE PATIENT DIAGNOSTIC STATEMENT

Identifying an incorrect nursing diagnosis or misstatement of problems/needs can lead to incorrect goals/outcomes and inappropriate nursing interventions. This can result in inappropriate/inadequate treatment of the patient that may not resolve the problem and that may, on occasion, place the nurse at risk for legal liability. When you have read through the items in this Box, proceed to Practice Activity 3–2.

- *Using the Medical Diagnosis:* Self-Care Deficit, related to stroke.
  Correct: Self-Care Deficit, related to neuromuscular impairment.
- *Relating the Problem to an Unchangeable Situation:* High risk for injury related to blindness.
  Correct: High risk for injury related to unfamiliarity with surroundings.
- *Confusing the Etiology or Signs/Symptoms for the Problem:* Postoperative lung congestion related to bedrest.
  Correct: Airway Clearance, ineffective, related to general weakness and immobility.
- *Use of a Procedure Instead of the "Human Response":* Catheterization related to urinary retention.
  Correct: Urinary Retention related to perineal swelling.
- *Lack of Specificity:* Constipation related to nutritional intake.
  Correct: Constipation related to inadequate dietary bulk and fluid intake.
- *Combining Two Nursing Diagnoses:* Anxiety and Fear related to separation from parents.
  Correct: Fear related to separation from parents, or Anxiety, moderate, related to change in environment and unmet needs.
- *Relating One Nursing Diagnosis to Another:* Coping, individual ineffective, related to anxiety.
  Correct: Anxiety, severe, related to change in role functioning and socioeconomic status.
- *Use of Judgmental/Value-Laden Language:* Pain, chronic, related to secondary/monetary gain.
  Correct: Pain, chronic, related to recurrent muscle spasms. Note: The patient's complaint is valid, but the issue of secondary gain may require additional assessment to choose appropriate interventions.
- *Making Assumptions:* Parenting, altered, high risk for, related to inexperience (new mother).
  Correct: Knowledge Deficit: Child care issues related to lack of previous experience, unfamiliarity with resources. *Author note:* The label "Knowledge Deficit" can have negative connotations for the patient and may result in defensive responses. The authors support the use of a substitute label, "Learning Need."
- *Writing a Legally Inadvisable Statement:* Skin Integrity, impaired, related to not being turned q 2 h.
  Correct: Skin Integrity, impaired, related to pressure and altered circulation. Note: If a patient complication occurs as a result of poor care/failure to meet standards of care, an incident report would be completed to document what happened.

BOX 3–9 APPLICABLE NURSING DIAGNOSES ASSOCIATED WITH SELECTED MEDICAL DISORDERS

This box demonstrates how possible nursing diagnoses may be linked to medical disorders. This kind of linkage is often presented as choices for selection by the nurse in a diagnostic database, in various types of clinical pocket manuals, or on preprinted care planning forms. Its purpose is to assist in rapidly identifying other applicable nursing diagnoses, based on the changing needs of the patient; and to support the development of a decisive plan of care.

Once appropriate nursing diagnoses have been selected, the nurse can more easily validate the Assessment and Diagnosis phases of the nursing process, facilitating efforts to individualize and refine a plan of care.

Because the nursing process is cyclical and ongoing, however, other nursing diagnoses may become appropriate, based on changing individual patient situations. Therefore, the nurse must continually assess, identify, and validate new problems and evaluate the effectiveness of subsequent care.

AIDS (Acquired Immune Deficiency Syndrome)

Infection, high risk for, * progression to sepsis/overgrowth related to suppressed inflammatory response and immunosuppression in combination with inadequate primary defenses and malnutrition.

Fluid Volume Deficit, high risk for, * related to excessive losses: copious diarrhea, profuse sweating, vomiting, hypermetabolic state, and fever; restricted intake: nausea and anorexia; lethargy.

Injury, high risk for, altered clotting factors, * related to decreased vitamin K absorption, alteration in hepatic function, presence of autoimmune antiplatelet antibodies, malignancies (Kaposi's sarcoma), and circulating endotoxins (sepsis).

Pain, related to tissue inflammation/destruction: infections, internal/external cutaneous lesions, rectal excoriation, malignancies, necrosis; myalgias and arthralgias, abdominal cramping evidenced by complaints of pain, self-focusing/narrowed focus, alteration in muscle tone, guarding behaviors, autonomic responses, and restlessness.

Skin Integrity, impaired, related to immunologic deficit (AIDS-related dermatitis, bacterial/fungal infections, opportunistic disease processes/Kaposi's sarcoma), decreased level of activity, altered sensation, skeletal prominence, altered metabolic state evidenced by skin lesions; ulcerations, decubitus ulcer formation.

Fatigue, related to decreased metabolic energy production, increased energy requirements (hypermetabolic state), overwhelming psychologic/emotional demands and increased body temperature evidenced by inability to maintain usual routines, decreased performance, lethargy/listlessness, and disinterest in surroundings.

Cholelithiasis

Pain, related to inflammation and distention of tissues evidenced by

(Continued)

BOX 3-9 APPLICABLE NURSING DIAGNOSES ASSOCIATED WITH SELECTED MEDICAL DISORDERS (*Continued*)

complaints, guarding/distraction behaviors, and autonomic responses (changes in vital signs).

Nutrition, altered, less than body requirements, related to inability to ingest/absorb adequate nutrients (food intolerance/pain, nausea/vomiting, anorexia) evidenced by aversion to food/decreased intake and weight loss.

Knowledge Deficit [learning need], related to lack of information about pathophysiology, therapy choices, and self-care needs evidenced by verbalization of concerns, questions, and recurrence of condition.

Depressive Disorders (Mood Disorders)
MAJOR DEPRESSION DYSTHYMIA

*Violence, high risk for, directed at self/others,** related to depressed mood and feelings of worthlessness and hopelessness.

Coping, ineffective, individual, related to personal vulnerability, inadequate support systems, unrealistic perceptions, multiple life changes, inadequate coping method, unmet expectations, and actual/perceived loss evidenced by perception of events and stressors in a manner that precipitates depressive episode, perception of areas in life as unfulfilled or as losses, denial of loss, verbalization of inability to cope or ask for help, expression of guilt, crying/labile affect, and chronic anxiety/depression.

Sleep Pattern Disturbance, related to biochemical alterations (decreased serotonin), unresolved fears and anxieties, and inactivity evidenced by difficulty in falling/remaining asleep, early morning awakening, complaints of not feeling well rested, dark circles under eyes.

* *Note:* A high risk diagnosis is not evidenced by signs and symptoms as the problem has not occurred and nursing interventions are directed at prevention.

Extracted from Doenges and Moorhouse: Nurse's Clinical Pocket Manual. FA Davis, Philadelphia, 1990.

IN A NUTSHELL . . .

How to Write a Patient Diagnostic Statement

1. Using physical assessment and history-taking interview techniques, collect both subjective and objective data from patient, significant other, family members, other healthcare professionals, and patient records. It is recommended that a nursing framework such as Diagnostic Divisions (Doenges and Moorhouse), Functional Health Patterns (Gordon), or Human Response Patterns (NANDA) be used to do this.

2. Organize the collected data using a nursing framework (see Item 1, above), a body systems approach (cardiovascular, gastrointestinal, etc.), a head-to-toe approach (head, neck, thorax, etc.), or a combination of these. Your institution may well use its own clustering model. If you have used a nursing framework, however, you will discover that information in the patient database is already conveniently structured for ease in identifying applicable nursing diagnoses.

3. Using diagnostic reasoning skills, review and analyze the database to identify cues (signs and symptoms) suggesting problems/needs which can be described by nursing diagnostic labels. Checking the NANDA definitions of specific diagnoses can be of further assistance in distinguishing between two or more potentially applicable labels (see Appendix A).

4. Consider alternative rationales for the identified cues by comparing and contrasting the relationships among and between data, and isolating etiologic factors. This will allow you to determine which nursing diagnosis label(s) may be most appropriate, while ruling out those which are not.

5. Test your selection of nursing diagnosis label(s) and associated etiology(ies) for appropriate "fit" by:
   - Confirming the NANDA nursing diagnosis and definition for your choice of diagnostic label **[P]**
   - Comparing your proposed etiology with the NANDA "Related Factors" or "Risk Factors" associated with that particular diagnosis **[E]**
   - Comparing your identified signs and symptoms or cues with the NANDA "Defining Characteristics" for the selected diagnosis **[S]**

6. Reevaluate your list of selected diagnoses to be sure that all patient problems/needs are accounted for. Then, order your list according to a needs priority model (the Maslow or Kalish models are usually used) and classify each diagnosis as *active* (signs and symptoms supporting it are already present), *high risk* (risk factors are present, but the problem has not yet occurred), or *resolved* (problem no longer requires nursing action).

7. Write the patient diagnostic statement for each diagnosis on your list. A 3-part statement using the P E S format will be needed for active diagnoses, and an adaptation of the P E S format will be used to create the 2-part statement needed for high risk diagnoses. Resolved diagnoses do not require diagnostic statements.

3-Part Patient Diagnostic Statement

To write the patient diagnostic statement for active diagnoses, combine (1) the confirmed nursing diagnosis label [P], (2) related factors [E], and (3) defining characteristics [S]. These elements are linked together by the phrases "related to" and "as evidenced by":

PROBLEM: [nursing diagnosis label]
ETIOLOGY: Related to [etiologic factors]
SIGNS AND SYMPTOMS: As evidenced by: [defining characteristics]

2-Part Diagnostic Statement

To write the diagnostic statement for high risk diagnoses, combine (1) the confirmed high risk nursing diagnosis label [P] and (2) the associated risk factors [E]. These elements are linked together by the phrase "related to":

PROBLEM: [high risk nursing diagnosis label]
ETIOLOGY: Related to [associated risk factors]

PRACTICE ACTIVITY 3-1

IDENTIFYING THE P E S COMPONENTS OF THE PATIENT DIAGNOSTIC STATEMENT

Instructions (questions 1-5): *Identify the P E S components of each of these diagnostic statements:*

1. Anxiety, severe, related to changes in health status of fetus/self and threat of death as evidenced by restlessness, tremors, focus on self/fetus.

   P = _____   E = _____

   S = _____

2. Thought Processes, altered, related to pharmacologic stimulation of the nervous system evidenced by altered attention span, disorientation, and hallucinations.

   P = _____   E = _____

   S = _____

3. Coping, individual, ineffective, related to maturational crisis evidenced by inability to meet role expectations and alcohol abuse.

   P = _____   E = _____

   S = _____

4. Hyperthermia related to increased metabolic rate and dehydration evidenced by elevated temperature, flushed skin, tachycardia, and tachypnea.

   P = _____   E = _____

   S = _____

5. Pain, acute, related to tissue distention and edema evidenced by verbal complaints, guarding behavior, and changes in vital signs.

   P = _____   E = _____

   S = _____

6. Explain the difference between active and high risk (potential) diagnoses:

   _____

   _____

7. Give an example of an active and a potential (high risk) problem for a patient with 2nd degree burns of the hand.

   _____

   _____

PRACTICE ACTIVITY 3-2

IDENTIFYING CORRECT AND INCORRECT PATIENT DIAGNOSTIC STATEMENTS

Label each patient diagnostic statement as correct or incorrect. Identify why a statement is incorrect:

1. Airway Clearance, ineffective, related to increased pulmonary secretions and bronchospasm

   evidenced by wheezing, tachypnea, and ineffective cough. _____

   _____

   _____

2. Thought Processes, altered, related to delusional thinking, poor reality base evidenced by

   persecutory thoughts of "I am victim," and interference with ability to think clearly and

   logically. _____

   _____

   _____

3. Gas Exchange, impaired, related to bronchitis evidenced by rhonchi, dyspnea, and cyanosis.

   _____

   _____

   _____

4. Knowledge Deficit, diabetic care, related to inaccurate follow-through of instructions evi-

   denced by information misinterpretation and lack of recall. _____

   _____

   _____

5. Pain [acute], related to tissue distention and edema evidenced by complaints of severe colicky

   pain in right flank, elevated pulse and respirations, and restlessness. _____

   _____

   _____

SUMMARY

Although identifying a correct nursing diagnosis requires *time* to analyze the gathered data and to validate the diagnosis, it is the pivotal part of the nursing process. The time taken to formulate a patient diagnostic statement and to plan care results in increased nursing efficiency, better use of time for all nursing staff, and the delivery of appropriate patient care.

Some nurses still organize care directly around medical diagnoses, spending the majority of their time following medical orders. The medical diagnosis has a narrower focus than that of nursing diagnoses, because it is based on pathology. A nursing diagnosis is more broad, taking into account the psychologic, social, spiritual (as well as physiologic) responses of the patient. NANDA diagnostic labels are most frequently used in formulating diagnostic statements which are structured in a three-part Problem, Etiology, and Signs/Symptoms (P E S) format (Appendix A). Two-part statements may be used for high risk or potential diagnoses.

At times, what appears easy to do in theory may be difficult to achieve in practice. Nurses often have visionary ideas for the delivery of quality care to all patients. All too frequently, turning those ideas into actions can seem to be a frustrating exercise in futility. However, as the nurse works and becomes more familiar with nursing diagnoses, the patient goals, related outcomes, and nursing interventions for attaining these goals become more readily apparent. Thus, accurate and complete nursing diagnoses form the basis for the activities of the Planning phase of the nursing process, discussed in Chapter 4.

WORK PAGE: Chapter Three

1. What is the definition of problem identification? _____

_____

2. What two factors influenced the development and acceptance of nursing diagnosis as the language

of nursing? _____

_____

_____

3. List three reasons for using nursing diagnosis:

a. _____

b. _____

c. _____

4. List the six steps of diagnostic reasoning:

a. _____

b. _____

c. _____

d. _____

e. _____

f. _____

5. Name the components of the Patient Diagnostic Statement:

a. _____

b. _____

c. _____

6. If a high risk or potential problem is identified, how is the Patient Diagnostic Statement altered?

_____

_____

7. What is the difference between a medical and a nursing diagnosis? _____

_____

_____

_____

8. Which of these patient diagnostic statements are stated correctly? Indicate by placing a C before correct statements. Differentiate actual (A) from high risk (HR) problems by placing an A or HR after each statement:

_____ Knowledge Deficit, drug therapy related to misinterpretation and unfamiliarity with resources as evidenced by request for information and statement of misconception. _____

_____ High Risk for Infection, related to altered lung expansion, decreased ciliary action, decreased hemoglobin, and invasive procedures. _____

_____ Urinary Elimination, altered related to indwelling catheter evidenced by inability to void. _____

_____ Anxiety, moderate related to change in health status, role functioning, and socioeconomic status evidenced by apprehension, insomnia, and feelings of inadequacy. _____

9. Underline the cues in the patient database below which indicate that a problem may exist, and write a Patient Diagnostic Statement based on your findings:

Vignette: Sally is visited by the Public Health Nurse for follow-up 6 days postdelivery. She complains about her bowels but says she has been drinking plenty of fluids, including fruit juices, and has been eating a balanced diet.

ELIMINATION SECTION FROM THE PATIENT DATABASE

Subjective

Usual bowel patterns: every morning   **Laxative use:** rare/MOM pm
Character of stool: brown, formed   **Last BM:** 3 days ago
History of bleeding: no   **Hemorrhoids:** last 5 weeks
Constipation: since delivery   **Diarrhea:** no
Usual voiding pattern: 3–4 x/day   **Incontinence:** no   **Urgency:** no
Character of urine: yellow   **Pain/burning/difficulty voiding:** no
History of kidney/bladder disease: several bladder infections, last one 6 years ago
Associated complaints: pain with stool, nausea, "I just can't go no matter what I do."

Objective

Abdomen tender: yes   **Soft/firm:** somewhat firm   **Palpable mass:** no
Size/girth: enlarged/postpartal
Bowel sounds: present all 4 quadrants but decreased
Hemorrhoids: visual examination not done.

Now, write the Patient Diagnostic Statement. Refer to the listing of Nursing Diagnoses in Appendix

A to compare diagnostic labels addressing bowel elimination. _____

_____

_____

_____

_____

_____

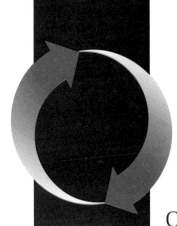

The Planning Phase: Creating the Plan of Care

ANA Standard 3: The plan of nursing care includes goals derived from the nursing diagnoses.

ANA Standard 4: The plan of nursing care includes the priorities and the prescribed nursing approaches or measures to achieve the goals derived from the nursing diagnoses.

As the etiology, signs, and symptoms previously identified and incorporated into the diagnostic statement are reviewed, the nurse's attention shifts to the Planning phase of the nursing process. Attention is now focused on the most appropriate actions which will effectively address the patient's prob-

PLAN OF CARE—
written evidence of
the second and third
steps of the Nursing
Process that identifies
the patient's
problems/needs,
goals/outcomes of
care, and interventions
to treat the
problems/needs.

PLANNING—the third
step of the Nursing
Process during which
goals/outcomes are
determined and
interventions chosen.

lems/needs. The nurse begins to set priorities; establish goals; identify desired outcomes; and determine specific nursing interventions. These actions are documented as the **PLAN OF CARE**, which then serves to guide the activities of all healthcare workers who are involved in the patient's care. Whenever possible, the patient and/or significant other(s) are included in the process of **PLANNING,** so that they may contribute to, participate in, and take responsibility for their own care and the achievement of the desired outcomes and goals.

SETTING PRIORITIES FOR PATIENT CARE

The starting point for the planning of care is the establishment of a general ranking of the patient's problems/needs, so that the nurse's attention and subsequent actions are properly focused. While there are many ways of prioritizing patient needs, one framework which has been found useful is a hierarchy developed by Abraham Maslow (Fig. 4–1). In 1943, Maslow theorized that human behavior is motivated by a hierarchy arranged from the most basic to progressively higher-level needs. Physiologic needs are generally considered as base-line survival needs because they must be met in order for life to continue. When these base-level needs (such as food, fluid, and oxygen) are not satisfied, it is difficult or impossible to meet higher-level needs. Once base-level needs are satisfied, however, it becomes possible for higher-level needs (such as love, belonging, and self-esteem) to be addressed.

Richard Kalish expanded the structure of Maslow's hierarchy and further subdivided it to indicate more specific need categories. This expanded hierarchy can help you, as a nurse, to more precisely identify and prioritize patient needs (Fig. 4–2). Failure to meet human needs at any level can dramatically interfere with a patient's overall progress. Clearly, it is difficult to use Active Listening techniques (meeting a higher-level patient need for self-esteem) to teach a patient who is choking (a basic need of survival) about maintaining a patent airway.

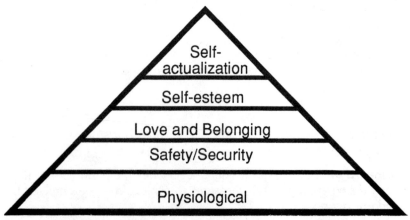

Figure 4–1 Maslow's hierarchy of needs. The pyramid of Maslow's hierarchy is a model which allows us to look at human behavior in a structured way, to determine physiologic and psychologic needs. Physiologic needs appear at the bottom or base of the pyramid. Maslow's theory tells us that these lower-level needs must be met before higher-level needs (such as Self-esteem) can be addressed. This knowledge of the needs that must be met first can help the nurse determine the priorities of patient care.

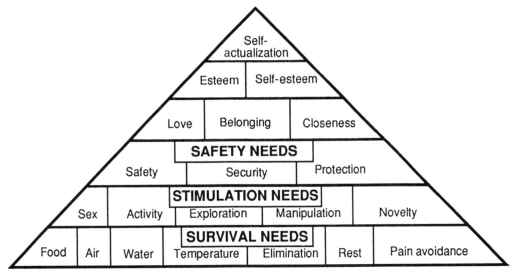

Figure 4–2 Kalish's expanded hierarchy. In an expansion of Maslow's model, Kalish restructured the first two levels of Maslow's pyramid (Physiologic and Safety/Security needs) into three levels and identified more-specific subcategories. The base level is labeled Survival, the second level Stimulation, and the third level Safety. The refinement of these subcategories can further assist the nurse to identify the priorities for planning patient care.

Once the priorities of care are determined, the patient's problems are then ranked, based on some system (such as Maslow's hierarchy) which can help the nurse to identify lower- to higher-level needs. This is necessary because it is usually extremely difficult to work with more than three to five patient problems at one time, depending on each problem's complexity. By ranking the patient's problems/needs, you can proceed in a logical way to facilitate your patient's recovery.

For example, basic survival needs (i.e., air, water, and food) must be met before other needs can be considered. Sample diagnostic labels involving basic survival needs include Airway Clearance, ineffective and Nutrition, altered, less than body requirements. Safety needs are next in order of importance. Nursing diagnostic labels relating to safety needs include Violence, high risk for, directed at self/others; Injury, high risk for; Health Maintenance, altered. Once these categories of needs are met, concerns regarding needs in the social, self-esteem, and self-actualization categories can be considered. Examples of nursing diagnosis labels relating to these categories of needs are: Social Interaction, impaired (a need for relationships with others); Self-Esteem, disturbance (the need to feel good about oneself); and Family Coping, potential for growth (a need for family and belonging). Practice Activity 4–1 will give you some experience prioritizing patient problems based on levels of need.

Establishing Patient Goals

Once patient problems have been prioritized, the **GOALS** for treatment/ discharge criteria are established. They are broadly stated and reflect the general direction toward which the patient is expected to progress.

GOALS—broad guidelines indicating the overall direction for movement as a result of the interventions of the healthcare team; divided into long-term goals and short-term goals.

PRACTICE ACTIVITY 4–1

PRIORITIZING NURSING DIAGNOSES

Instructions: Prioritize these three sets of nursing diagnoses using a ranking system with 1 as the most basic or more immediate underlying need.

a. _____ Incontinence, stress

_____ Sexuality Patterns, altered

_____ Airway Clearance, ineffective

_____ Skin Integrity, impaired, high risk

b. _____ Gas Exchange, impaired

_____ Knowledge Deficit

_____ Hypothermia

_____ Infection, high risk for

c. _____ Pain, acute

_____ Self-Esteem, chronic low

_____ Physical Mobility, impaired

_____ Social Isolation

Short-term and Long-term Goals

LONG-TERM GOALS
—those goals that may not be achieved prior to discharge from care but require continued attention by patient and/or others, as indicated.

SHORT-TERM GOALS
—those goals that usually must be met prior to discharge or movement to a less acute level of care.

Goals involve varying timeframes and may be either long-term or short-term. **LONG-TERM GOALS** indicate the overall direction/end result of care and may very well <u>not</u> be achieved prior to discharge. Examples of long-term goals might be "Maintains control of blood sugar level" or "Uses resources/supports to prevent rehospitalization." **SHORT-TERM GOALS** are more specific guides for care and must usually be met <u>prior</u> to discharge or transfer to a less acute level of care, supervision, or support. Depending upon the patient's anticipated length of stay/care, a short-term goal may be evaluated within a few hours or over the period of several therapeutic sessions. This period of time could reflect as much as several calendar weeks, if the patient is seen for counseling/therapy on a weekly, or even monthly, basis. Examples of short-term goals might be "Reduces myocardial workload" or "Maintains impulse control."

If the short-term goal is to be met within the nursing shift during which it is identified, the goal need not be written on the plan of care but *would* be noted in the progress note. If the goal is not accomplished by the end of the shift, it would then be added to the plan of care, with a new timeframe, so that oncoming nurses can continue to work toward the goal.

IDENTIFYING DESIRED OUTCOMES

The next step in developing the plan of care is the formation of specific, measurable **OUTCOMES**, which are defined as patient responses that are achievable, that are desired by the patient, and that can be attained within a defined time period given the present situation and resources. These desired outcomes are the measurable steps toward achieving the patient goals which were established earlier. Because they must be measurable, outcome statements need to:

- be specific
- be realistic
- consider the patient's circumstances and desires
- indicate a definite timeframe for achievement
- provide measurable evaluation criteria for determination of success or failure in achieving the desired effect

OUTCOME—the result of actions undertaken to achieve a broader goal; measurable steps to achieve the goals of treatment and to meet discharge criteria.

Desired outcomes are written by listing items/behaviors which can be observed and monitored to determine whether or not a positive/acceptable outcome has been achieved within the indicated timeframe. For example, "Verbalizes understanding of disease process and potential complications. . . . " This itemized listing of outcomes then serves as the evaluation tool and will be discussed more fully in Chapter 6. Take a moment to look over Box 4–1 to give you a better idea of how to make the distinction between goals and outcomes.

Measurable action verbs are used to describe outcomes. For instance, "Patient will: <u>ambulate</u> with use of cane." Some examples of this type of verb are: discusses, states, identifies, administers, explains, and reports. Refer to Box 4–2 for additional examples. Passive words are generally avoided.

The use of specific time elements in outcome statements also provide measurable criteria, such as "Patient will: ambulate with cane without assistance <u>within 3 days</u>." On occasion, some outcomes may be ongoing because they do not have a specific timeframe, short of discharge from care. Examples of these ongoing outcomes would be statements such as "Patient will: maintain a patent airway" or "Patient will: be free of skin breakdown." Each of these situations will be monitored by the nurse and any patient findings documented regularly. However, the situations may not be <u>resolved</u> until the patient's condition/status changes or discharge has occurred.

When outcomes are properly written, they provide direction for the nurse in planning and validating the choice of appropriate nursing interventions.

For example:

- Patient will: identify individual nutritional needs within 30 hours.
- Patient will: formulate a dietary plan based on these needs within 48 hours.

From these desired outcomes, the nurse knows that the patient's level of dietary knowledge should be assessed, individual patient needs identified, and patient teaching information presented to provide the patient with the tools necessary to formulate a dietary plan.

Remember, though, interventions can be wide-ranging. The outcome statement "Patient will: verbalize acceptance of actual body image within 2

BOX 4-1 DISTINGUISHING BETWEEN GOALS AND OUTCOMES

Goals are overall, broad directions to guide the plan of care. A broad *goal* for a patient with chronic obstructive pulmonary disease (COPD) might be:

- Ventilation/oxygenation adequate to allow a functional lifestyle.

Outcomes are the desired results of actions undertaken to achieve the broader *goal* and are the measurable steps to achieving the *goals* of treatment/discharge criteria. Often there is more than one *outcome* for each *goal*. The integral *outcomes* to achieve the above *goal* could include:

- Maintains patent airway with breath sounds clear.
- Demonstrates techniques to improve airway clearance, i.e., use of pursed-lip breathing, liquefying secretions, and/or nebulizer therapy.
- Initiates necessary lifestyle changes and participates in treatment regimen.

BOX 4-2 ACTION VERBS USEFUL IN WRITING MEASURABLE OUTCOMES

The following are examples of action verbs that can be measured or observed. Using action rather than "passive" verbs provides a means by which patient progress can be determined.

> List, Record, Name, State
> Describe, Explain, Identify
> Demonstrate, Use, Schedule
> Differentiate, Compare, Relate
> Design, Prepare, Formulate
> Select, Choose, Compare
> Increase/Decrease, Stand, Walk, Participate

For example: The patient will: List three things he understands about his diagnosis. The patient will: Walk to the end of the hall and back three times today.

Below are a few samples of "passive" verbs. Notice that the "actions" described by the verbs are not measurable:

> Understand, Feel, Learn, Know, Accept

For example: The patient will: Understand his treatment plan. How will the nurse measure achievement and know that the patient understands?

weeks" may call for interventions ranging from learning to recognize and express own feelings about body changes to developing a program of diet and exercise to promote weight loss, to instruction in the use of makeup, hairstyles, and ways of dressing that maximize figure assets.

All outcomes should tell the readers specifically what the patient is working on or doing. If the outcome does not seem to logically relate to the goals for treatment/discharge, it should be questioned. Is the outcome, in fact, a valid component of the plan of care? With this in mind, there is a simple and straightforward method of determining whether or not an outcome is correctly written: Just ask yourself if you could *observe* the patient in the performance of the behavior indicated. If the answer is no, the desired, measurable outcome you have written should be modified. Below are several pairs of correctly and incorrectly written outcomes with notations to identify the desired elements. When you have finished looking them over, work through the exercises in Practice Activity 4–2.

1. **Incorrect:** "Understands insulin therapy within 48 hours."
    or
    "Explains reasons for the steps of insulin administration within 48 hours."
    > *Rationale:* This patient outcome states a clear time line, but can you measure a patient "understanding"? This outcome needs a measurable action verb.

    Correct: "Demonstrates correct insulin administration techniques within 48 hours."
    > *Rationale:* These are well-written outcomes that are observable, measurable, and time limited.

2. **Incorrect:** "Requires no reminders from staff regarding dietary restrictions within 3 days."
    > *Rationale:* This outcome tells what the *staff* will do, not what the patient will do.

    Correct: "Lists individual dietary restrictions and makes appropriate choices from daily menu within 3 days."
    > *Rationale:* This outcome is observable and easy to document.

3. **Incorrect:** "Receives fewer restrictions for defying staff instructions during the next 2 weeks."
    > *Rationale:* What exactly is the definition of "fewer"? A specific number is better. What constitutes "defiance," and what is the patient *doing*? According to this outcome, the patient "receives" fewer restrictions, which places the patient in an essentially passive role. Good measurable outcomes state what the patient actively does.

    Correct: "Decreases infractions of rules from the current rate of five per week to no more than two per week within 7 days."
    > *Rationale:* Incidents of violation of unit rules are events which are observable, well documented, and easy to track. This is also time limited and is a well-written outcome.

PRACTICE ACTIVITY 4–2

IDENTIFYING CORRECTLY STATED OUTCOMES

Instructions: Identify which of the following outcome statements are correct, and modify those that are not.

1. Patient will: List individual risk factors and appropriate interventions. _____

    _____

2. Patient will: Identify adaptive/protective measures for individual situation by discharge.

    _____

3. Patient will: Understand behaviors, lifestyle changes necessary to promote physical safety

    within 72 hours. _____

    _____

4. Airway is patent, aspiration is prevented, ongoing. _____

    _____

5. Patient will: Assume responsibility for own learning by using available resources and partici-

    pating in group discussions within 3 days. _____

    _____

SELECTING APPROPRIATE NURSING INTERVENTIONS

Nursing interventions are prescriptions for specific behaviors expected from the patient, and actions to be carried out by nurses. The expectation is that the prescribed behavior/actions will benefit the patient and/or significant other(s) in a predictable way, related to the identified problem/need and chosen outcomes. These interventions have the intent of individualizing care and are geared toward meeting a specific patient need. They should be age/situation appropriate and promote identified patient strengths, when possible.

For example:

- *Discussion of fears* may help to reduce the adult patient's level of anxiety, while an infant will respond more positively to *holding and cuddling.*
- Orange juice is a good choice for fluid replacement *unless* the patient has open lesions on the oral mucosa, in which case, mild fruit nectars would be preferred, as acidic juices will cause pain.

- The patient demonstrates strong creative abilities, so you instruct the patient in the use of visualization to help with stress reduction and pain management.

When identifying nursing interventions, the body of scientific knowledge (rationale) that supports these interventions must be known, because the nurse is accountable for being current and accurate. **NURSING STANDARDS** and agency policy must also be considered when choosing specific interventions. The interventions must be deliberate and purposeful and include independent nursing activities (such as monitoring/focused assessments, counseling, and teaching), as well as any collaborative activities necessary to carry out orders from other healthcare providers (including consultation by and referral to other providers).

Nursing interventions should be specific and clearly state:

- the date the intervention is written
- an action verb reflecting the activity to be performed
- qualifiers of how, when, where, time/frequency, and amount
- signature and/or initials of originating nurse

For example:

- 1/27 Assist as needed with self-care activities each AM. *A G*
- 6/12 Record respiratory and pulse rates before, during, and after activity. *CＯ*
- 3/13 Inspect wound during each dressing change. *MB*
- 10/12 Measure intake and output hourly. *SＬ*

Note: When the original plan of care is written, a single date and signature are sufficient. As subsequent interventions are added, they should be individually dated and initialed. Box 4–3 is an example which walks you through the first three steps of the nursing process. Patient data are presented, and a patient problem is identified. Then a goal, outcomes, and appropriate interventions are chosen to treat the problem.

NURSING STANDARD —*identified criterion against which nursing care is compared and evaluated; generally reflects the minimum level for nursing care.*

THE PATIENT PLAN OF CARE

Planning care can save valuable time when the goals of care, patient outcomes, and nursing interventions to achieve them are clearly identified, and then recorded, for all to see. The documentation of the planning process is the patient's plan of care, which some nurses refer to as the "care plan." This plan of care is written to:

- *provide continuity of care* from nurse to nurse, from nursing shift to nursing shift, or even from one unit/care setting to another
- *enhance communication* as the written plan becomes a permanent part of the patient record and supplies consistent information for each person who reads it
- *assist with the determination of agency or unit staffing needs*, setting priorities for the shift work schedule, and individual patient assignments
- *support documentation of the nursing process* by providing reminders of what needs to be charted and when evaluations should be done

PRACTICE ACTIVITY 4-3

IDENTIFYING CORRECTLY STATED INTERVENTIONS

Instructions: Identify which of the following interventions are correctly stated, and rewrite those that are not.

1. Walk length of hall 2×/day with assistance of two staff members. _____

   _____

   _____

2. Force fluids. _____

   _____

   _____

3. Pericare after each BM. _____

   _____

   _____

4. Encourage deep breathing exercises and cough q 2 h. _____

   _____

   _____

5. Reduce environmental stimuli. _____

   _____

   _____

6. Provide written handout for side-effects of medications prior to discharge. _____

   _____

- ***serve as a teaching tool*** that supports the sharing of nurses' expertise and fosters professional growth as nurses learn what interventions are successful

The fields of nursing and medicine are closely interrelated and have implications for each other. This close relationship includes the exchange of data, the sharing of ideas/thinking, and the development of a plan of care that includes all data pertinent to the individual patient/family/significant other(s). The same type of relationship also extends to all healthcare disciplines which have contact with the patient.

Because of this relationship, the plan of care contains more than simply the actions initiated by medical orders (collaborative actions). It also contains a combination of nursing orders (independent actions) as well and is the written coordination of care given by all health-related disciplines. The nurse becomes the person responsible for seeing to it that all of these different activities are coordinated into a functional whole. This coordination of the efforts of caregivers is essential to delivering holistic, cost-effective health care which promotes optimal patient recovery in a timely manner.

As a student, exercises in "care planning" are assigned to allow you to demonstrate your mastery of the nursing process and your application of related knowledge from other science disciplines. The need to identify and prepare for every possible patient problem in a given situation results in the creation of a *case study*, instead of the more abbreviated and succinct plan of care that is usually found in the nursing unit Kardex in most hospitals. However, the length of time and degree of detail required to complete these "case studies" often cause nursing students to develop a negative attitude toward planning care. It is important to keep this activity in perspective, for as a professional nurse, you will need to plan care for your patients on a daily basis. Mastery of the skills of planning care will allow you to complete this activity in a timely fashion.

The plan of care is primarily a communication tool which directs the patient's care. However, newly formulated requirements of outside agencies (for example, **JCAHO**, medicare, private insurance companies) stipulate that the nurse is to be responsible for the planning of patient care. In addition, this plan of care is to be documented in the patient's record. For these reasons, the plan of care is now a permanent part of the patient's record, since it contains the *outline* for the care provided.

JCAHO—*Joint Commission on Accreditation of Healthcare Organizations; surveying body which certifies clinical and organization performance of an institution following established guidelines.*

DISCHARGE PLANNING

As you plan for the patient's present needs, you must also consider future needs, especially eventual discharge from the healthcare facility. Discharge planning begins upon entry into the healthcare setting, is crucial to assure continuity of care, and includes the anticipated discharge destination (e.g., home or skilled nursing facility). The nurse is committed to planning continuity of care between nursing personnel, between services within the care setting, and between the care setting and the community. The nurse may also be responsible for initiating/cooperating in referrals to other community services, providing needed direction for patient/family who are learning to facilitate recovery and promote wellness.

DOCUMENTING THE PLAN OF CARE

The plan of care may be recorded on a single page or in a multiple-page format—such as one page for each diagnostic statement for a particular patient. The page (or pages) may be kept in a folder (Kardex) at the nursing station, in the patient's chart, or at the bedside to communicate and provide direction on a daily basis.

The format for documenting the plan of care is determined by agency policy. Student plans of care are individually generated and very detailed. As a practicing professional, you might well use a computer with a care plan database, or standardized care plan forms, reflecting the basic nursing standards of care to which personal patient data, nonroutine care, and qualifiers such as time or amount are added, as appropriate. For example:

Measure intake and output [*insert frequency*]
Increase oral fluids [*insert amount and frequency*]
Medicate with [*insert name of medication, dose, and frequency*] for pain
Weigh with bedscale [*insert time, frequency*]

Some computerized systems for plans of care generate an updated plan at the beginning of each shift. The care provided during the new shift is then recorded directly to the online plan of care throughout that shift. This format serves the dual purpose of documenting both the planning and implementation steps of the nursing process, and of continually updating the plan of care and the patient's record.

As previously noted, the plan of care is the visualization of the nursing process. As such, it is preserved as part of the patient's permanent record. Therefore, all entries need to be dated and initialed or signed. Use key words instead of complete sentences, only approved abbreviations/symbols, and with referral to procedure manuals as appropriate.

For example:

- 8/15 Routine urinary catheter care q shift. *DS*
- 9/2 NPO after 6 AM, 9/13. *JD*
- 3/7 Maintain subarachnoid bolt per protocol. *SP*

Regardless of the format used, the plan of care contains identifying patient data (including medical diagnosis), patient diagnostic statements, goals/outcomes, interventions as well as providing space to record the status of the outcomes (i.e., achieved, revised, or deleted) as shown in Figure 4–3.

VALIDATING THE PLAN OF CARE

Before the plan of care is implemented, it should be reviewed to assure that:

- It is based on accepted nursing practice reflecting knowledge of scientific principles, nursing standards of care, and agency policies.
- It provides for the safety of the patient in that the care provided will do no harm.
- The patient diagnostic statements are supported by the patient data.
- The goals and outcomes are measurable/observable and can be achieved.
- The interventions can benefit the patient/significant other(s) in a predictable way to achieve the identified outcomes and are arranged in a logical sequence, as appropriate.
- It demonstrates individualized patient care by inclusion of patient and

Patient: Donald   Age: 46   DOB: 2/4/44   Sex: M   Admission: 11/12/90 - 15:40   Dx: Acute Anxiety

Date:	Patient Diagnostic Statement	Goal	Interventions	Outcomes	Status
11/12 Problem #5	Coping, individual ineffective related to situational crisis of unemployment, personal vulnerability evidenced by reported inability to cope, use of alcohol, insomnia and diminished problem-solving.	short term: managing own situation effectively long term: actively seeking employment and expresses sense of self-worth.	1. Assess level of anxiety and Donald's perception of situation 2. Note verbal/nonverbal behaviors of anxiety 3. Look in q 2 hr and PRN 4. Encourage verbalization, expression of feelings of denial/depression/anger 5. Discuss normalcy of these feelings 6. Identify current coping mechanisms 7. Note effectiveness/need for change 8. Discuss/refer to resources: social worker, alcohol counselor, support group, AA	Verbalizes awareness of sources of anxiety (1600 11/14) Demonstrates congruency between feelings/behavior (1600 11/15) Demonstrates initial problem-solving skills (1600 11/15) Identifies options and resources available for assistance (1600 11/16)	Achieved 11/14 1630 R.S. Achieved 11/15 1600 P.D. Achieved 11/15 1600 P.D. Achieved 11/15 1600 P.D.

Figure 4–3   Sample documentation of a plan of care.

significant other(s) concerns, physical and psychosocial needs, and capabilities.

PROFESSIONAL CONCERNS RELATED TO THE PLAN OF CARE

Professional concerns associated with the identification of patient problems/needs in the construction of the plan of care are:

- What is the nurse's responsibility once a nursing diagnosis is made if the patient is discharged from care before all short-term outcomes are met and/or problems are resolved?
- Whose responsibility is it for follow-through for provision and evaluation of care once discharge has occurred?
- Who is responsible for monitoring patient progress toward long-term outcomes?
- Should this information be shared with the patient's admitting/primary physician or office nurse?
- Is the nurse who has made a nursing diagnosis responsible for follow-through to its resolution?

PRACTICE ACTIVITY 4–4

DOCUMENTING THE PLAN OF CARE

Instructions: Record the plan of care information from Box 4–3 on pages 75–76 using the following documentation format.

DATE	PATIENT DIAGNOSTIC STATEMENT	GOAL	INTERVENTIONS	OUTCOMES	STATUS

BOX 4–3 APPLICATION OF THE NURSING PROCESS THROUGH THE PLANNING PHASE

Phase I: Assessment

On 3/11/90 at 5:30 PM, Mike, a 20-year-old male (DOB 3/2/70), is admitted with a compound multiple fracture of the right tibia and fibula following a motorcycle accident.

ASSESSMENT DATA

Pain/Comfort

Subjective

Location: R lower leg   **Intensity (1–10):** 9   **Frequency:** since accident   **Quality:** sharp ache   **Duration:** constant
Radiation: Into knee   **Precipitation factors:** movement
How relieved: MS in ER   **Associated symptoms:** muscle spasms

Objective

Facial grimacing: Yes   **Guarding affected area:** Yes
Emotional response: stoic   **Narrowed focus:** Yes

Phase II: Problem Identification

Based on this assessment (and additional data recorded in other sections of the History Tool), using the diagnostic reasoning process and working with Appendix A, you choose the nursing diagnosis label "Pain, acute," and write the diagnostic statement:

   3/11/90   4 PM
   Patient Diagnostic Statement: Pain, acute, related to movement of bone fragments, soft tissue injury and edema evidenced by verbal complaints, guarding, muscle tension, and tachycardia.

Phase III: Planning

Goal: Pain free or controlled.
Outcomes:
   Patient will:

• Verbalize relief of pain within 30 minutes of administration of medication.
• Use relaxation skills to reduce level of pain by 3/12, 9 AM.
• Identify methods that provide relief by 3/12, 4 PM.

Interventions:

• Maintain limb rest of R leg × 24 hours.
• Elevate lower leg with folded blanket.
• Apply ice to area 20 min on/20 min off, as tolerated × 48 hours.
• Place cradle over foot of bed.

(Continued)

> **BOX 4–3 APPLICATION OF THE NURSING PROCESS THROUGH THE PLANNING PHASE (Continued)**
>
> • Document complaints and characteristics of pain.
> • Medicate with Demerol 75 mg and Vistaril 25 mg IM q 4 h, prn.
> • Demonstrate/encourage use of progressive relaxation techniques, deep breathing exercises and visualization.
> • Provide alternate comfort measures, position change, backrub.
>
> *S. Hunter RN*

Nationally, these issues are unresolved, and patient outcomes may remain unmet. Ethically, it is up to the nursing community and the healthcare industry to formulate policies that will promote optimum patient recovery and health maintenance. As a healthcare professional, you need to consider these issues as they will impact the care you provide, and you must develop the plan of care for your patient with these considerations in mind.

SUMMARY

Planning, setting goals, and choosing appropriate interventions are essential to the delivery of quality nursing care. These nursing activities comprise the Planning phase of the Nursing Process, and are documented in the plan of care for a particular patient. As a part of the patient's permanent record, the plan of care not only provides a means for the nurse who is actively caring for the patient to be aware of the problems (nursing diagnoses), goals, and actions to be taken, but it also substantiates the plan of care for third-party payers, accreditation, and legal needs.

Healthcare providers have a responsibility for planning with the patient and family for continuation of care to the eventual outcome of an optimal state of wellness or a dignified death. In the next chapter, you will have an opportunity to see how the plan of care can be implemented, prioritizing the interventions selected during the Planning phase to achieve the outcomes you identified for meeting short- and long-term patient goals.

WORK PAGE: Chapter Four

1. List three reasons why the plan of care is important:

a. _____

b. _____

c. _____

2. Briefly explain why setting priorities is necessary: _____

_____

_____

_____

3. What is the difference between a goal and an outcome? _____

_____

_____

_____

4. Identify five necessary components of patient outcomes:

a. _____   b. _____   c. _____

d. _____   e. _____

5. List four types of information that nursing interventions should contain:

a. _____

b. _____

c. _____

d. _____

6. Explain the difference between a measurable and a nonmeasurable verb and give an example of

each: _____

_____

_____

7. When does discharge planning begin? _____

_____

8. How is the plan of care documented? _____

_____

9. Identify two additional problems facing Mike, then set a goal with one outcome and two interventions for each problem.

> **Vignette:** Mike, the 20-year-old male with a compound fracture of the right lower leg, has other problems in addition to Pain, acute, previously discussed.
>
> His wound was contaminated by dirt and, although it was flushed with sterile saline solution before being packed and dressed, a cast was not applied because of tissue swelling and concerns about the wound. Instead, an external fixation device (a metal frame with pins extending through the skin and bone) is currently being used for immobilization of the tibia and fibula. The device is heavy and difficult for Mike to move without causing increased pain, and he is to remain on bedrest for 24 hours. In addition, IV antibiotics are to be administered q 4 h.

a. Problem: _____

_____

Goal: _____

Outcome: _____

Intervention:

1. _____

2. _____

b. Problem: _____

_____

Goal: _____

Outcome: _____

Intervention:

1. _____

2. _____

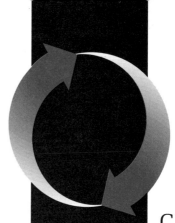

CHAPTER 5

The Implementation Phase: Putting the Plan of Care into Action

ANA Standard 5: Nursing actions provide for client/patient participation and health promotion, maintenance, and restoration.

ANA Standard 6: Nursing actions assist the client/patient to maximize his health capabilities.

IMPLEMENT/ IMPLEMENTATION— fourth step of Nursing Process in which the plan of care is put into action; performing identified interventions/ activities.

At this point of the nursing process, the nurse is ready to perform the interventions and activities recorded in the patient's plan of care. In order to **IMPLEMENT** this plan in a timely and cost-effective manner, the nurse first identifies the priorities for providing patient care. Then, as care is provided, data on the patient's response to each of the interventions are monitored. This information is documented, communicated to other healthcare providers as appropriate, and then used in evaluating and revising the plan of care in the following step of the nursing process (see Chapter 6).

IDENTIFYING CAREGIVING PRIORITIES

Regardless of how well a plan of care has been constructed, it cannot predict everything that will occur with a particular patient on a daily basis. The nurse's individual knowledge base, expertise, and recognition of agency routines allows her or him to exhibit the flexibility necessary to adapt to the changing needs of the patient. While listening closely to the change-of-shift report, the nurse will get the first clues about where to begin. On a worksheet such as the one shown in Fig. 5–1 or other form supplied by the agency, the nurse records specific information, interventions, or activities that are sequential or time related. Also, the plan of care is reviewed for outcomes that are to be evaluated during the shift and for routine procedures/treatments and medication administration.

Following completion of the shift report, a base-line assessment of each patient provides clues as to general physical status, equipment/supply needs, and safety concerns [e.g., patency of invasive lines (catheters/tubes) and IV flow rate]. At this time the nurse may recognize a change in the significance or severity of a patient problem which could affect the plan of care.

> **For example:** Robert, who is being treated for pneumonia, appears slightly cyanotic, at 7:30 AM. You will need to do a more thorough evaluation now to determine his immediate needs. This could include obtaining an arterial blood gas and restarting supplemental oxygen. In addition, you may decide against getting Robert up in a chair to eat his breakfast. Thus, interventions previously identified are not appropriate at this time, and new or alternate interventions are needed.

Pt.	7	8	9	10	11	12	1	2	3	Comments
Rbt		Vital signs Chair	Med	Bed bath	IV	V.S. Chair	Med	I & O		

Figure 5–1 Sample worksheet for the 7 AM to 3 PM shift. While listening to the change-of-shift report, you review the plan of care and begin to plan how you will implement specific interventions. You notice that Robert is to eat meals sitting up in a chair; therefore, he should be helped out of bed before the meal trays arrive on the unit. You identify times for medications, time for expected change of the IV bottle, and the routine time for calculating the intake and output for the shift. In addition, you are aware that Robert's family usually visits at lunch time, so you schedule hygiene needs appropriately while allowing Robert rest periods between activities.

This is also the time to review the plan of care with the patient/significant other to schedule activities and verify the patient's responsibilities.

> **For example:** Martha, a 52-year-old woman who had her gallbladder removed 3 days ago, will be able to bathe herself with limited assistance but would like to wait until after her physician has visited. Knowing that Dr. Jefferson usually makes rounds by 9:30 AM, you agree to a tentative bathing time of 10:00 AM.

Finally, legal and ethical concerns related to the interventions need to be considered. The wishes of the patient and family/significant other(s) regarding what is being done need to be discussed and respected.

> **For example:** Robert and his family have decided that if he should suffer respiratory failure, he is not to be placed on a respirator. This does not negate the need for intervention when you notice that he is developing problems but means you still need to act promptly to prevent/limit further deterioration. Therefore, in addition to providing oxygen and assessing breath sounds and airway patency, the head of Robert's bed is elevated, Robert is encouraged to deep-breathe and cough regularly, and other healthcare providers are notified as appropriate (e.g., physician and respiratory therapist).

Take a few minutes to work through Practice Activity 5–1 before continuing with the next section.

DELIVERING NURSING CARE

There are many activities ranging from simple tasks to complex procedures which can be involved in carrying out interventions to provide planned patient care. These activities may require direct "hands-on" care (such as a complete bed bath) or may merely require assisting a patient by setting up a pan of water and washing his back. Other activities often include instructing a patient/significant other regarding the management of their own care and then supervising their efforts. The patient and/or significant other(s) may need to be counseled regarding psychosocial concerns, treatment regimens, or alternative ways to manage healthcare needs. Throughout these activities, the nurse also monitors the patient and related resources (such as diagnostic studies and/or progress reports from other healthcare providers) for changes in health status/development of complications.

Before implementing the interventions listed in the plan of care, the nurse needs to be sure she or he:

- **Understands the reason for doing the intervention, its expected effect, and any potential hazards that can occur.** Without this knowledge, the nurse cannot be sure that the intervention will be beneficial. In addition, it will be difficult to determine if the desired effect is being achieved or if adaptations are required to provide for specific patient needs/safety concerns.

  > **For example:** The realizations that an arterial blood gas (ABG) study will provide information about Robert's current oxygenation status/needs and that supplemental oxygen will

PRACTICE ACTIVITY 5-1

SETTING YOUR WORK SCHEDULE FOR IMPLEMENTING THE PLAN OF CARE

Vignette: Martha had her gallbladder surgically removed 3 days ago. In reviewing the plan of care, you note the following:
- Obtain daily weight in gown and robe, 7:30 AM.
- Assist with bath/shower.
- Calculate I & O every 8 hours (6 AM–2 PM–10 PM).
- Change dressing twice a day and prn.
- Assess vital signs every 4 hours (8 AM–12 noon).
- Oral medications 9 AM–1 PM.
- Up in chair with meals.

1. Organize the above interventions and activities on the worksheet below:

Worksheet

Pt.	7	8	9	10	11	12	1	2	3	Comments

2. During nursing rounds, just after the change-of-shift report, you find Martha has been incontinent of urine. How will this affect your work plan? _____

_____

_____

_____

increase his oxygen level would be reasons for implementing these interventions in a slightly different sequence. The diagnostic study (ABG) should be obtained <u>before</u> the supplemental oxygen is begun, so that test results are not affected by the additional oxygen.

- **Provides an environment or milieu conducive to carrying out the planned interventions.** What is happening in the patient's environment is known to affect the person's physical and psychologic self (e.g., noise, temperature, activities).

> **For example:** Exposing Robert for a bed bath when the room is cold can cause him physical discomfort, as well as affect his psychologic response. Or, it is difficult for Martha to focus on your instructions for administering medications when the volume of the roommate's TV is turned up and visitors are talking loudly.

- **Consider which interventions can be combined to facilitate accomplishing the activities within your time constraints.** In some cases, shortcuts may be chosen or activities combined as long as consideration is given to the successful accomplishment of the outcome.

> **For example:** While administering medication to Robert at 1:00 PM, you can review the drug's actions, side-effects, and adverse reactions. Or, while assisting Martha with her bath, you may choose to discuss her concerns about caring for herself once she is discharged.

As noted in Box 5–1, one "simple" intervention such as providing a bedpan for a patient actually encompasses multiple nursing activities that, when listed individually, may appear to take considerable time and energy to perform. Careful prioritization of interventions and sequencing of related activities will help to accomplish these within what is actually a short period of time.

ONGOING DATA COLLECTION

Once the plan of care has been determined and put into action, the nurse monitors the patient to collect additional data. Talk to the patient, note changes in tone of voice and expression; or notice a reddened area on the coccyx as a backrub is provided. All of these data need to be noted, and their meaning validated. This information will be used to make decisions regarding the need for new goals, outcomes, interventions, and reprioritizing the plan of care during the evaluation process.

Documentation

It is legally required that all healthcare settings document nursing observations, the care provided, and the patient's response. This record serves as a communication tool and a resource to aid in determining the effectiveness of care and to assist in setting priorities for ongoing care. In order to simplify record keeping and to promote timely and accurate charting, many agencies use flow sheets to document routine activities, monitoring, and patient care (Fig. 5–2). Flow sheets reduce the need to write detailed progress notes. Instead, only variations from the recorded baseline and exceptions requiring more explanation are written in the progress note. Additional discussion about documentation and the use of progress notes will be presented in Chapter 7.

BOX 5–1 THE TRUTH ABOUT BEDPANS

Even the simplest of nursing tasks is really a complex series of actions and judgments, requiring professional knowledge and experience in order to provide optimal patient care.* Read through the short article reprinted below. You'll be interested to see just how complicated supplying a patient with a bedpan can be.

"There are many nursing activities interwoven in the 'simple' act of providing a bedpan. As a nurse, you assess the patient's:

> level of consciousness and mood, including self-image while dependent with these bodily functions.
>
> skin color, temperature, and suppleness.
>
> respiratory pattern and rate, breath sounds, and dyspnea with or without activity.
>
> comfort level with voiding or with stool.
>
> range of motion, strength, and any pain with movement.
>
> urine for color, amount odor, and by-products such as mucus or blood.
>
> stool for color, consistency, amount, and by-products such as mucus, undigested food, or blood.

You also determine

> if urine assessment relates to medications (Lasix, Pyridium, aminoglycosides), fluid intake, disease process (diabetes, dehydration, renal failure), or infection.
>
> if stool assessment relates to medication (antibiotics, barium enema, narcotics), food or fluid intake, disease process (cholelithiasis, Crohn's disease, bleeding ulcers), infection, activity or inactivity.
>
> if assessment demands any action and whether the doctor needs to be notified.

You then go on to teach:

> symptoms to watch for, comfort measures, and ways to maintain or achieve normal functioning.
>
> disease process and how it affects the individual.

On top of all that you:

> promote self-esteem by using proper technique, including disposal of waste material.
>
> obtain necessary specimens using correct procedure and send to lab.
>
> make sure patient is clean and dry to promote good skin integrity.
>
> model good handwashing technique upon completion.

* "The Truth about Bedpans" by Karen Tolin, RN, Joplin, MO, printed by *RN Magazine*.

Verbal Communication with the Healthcare Team

In addition to the written record, patient information is shared verbally with other healthcare providers. Whether reporting to another nurse, reviewing with a physician, or discussing with other resources (e.g., social worker,

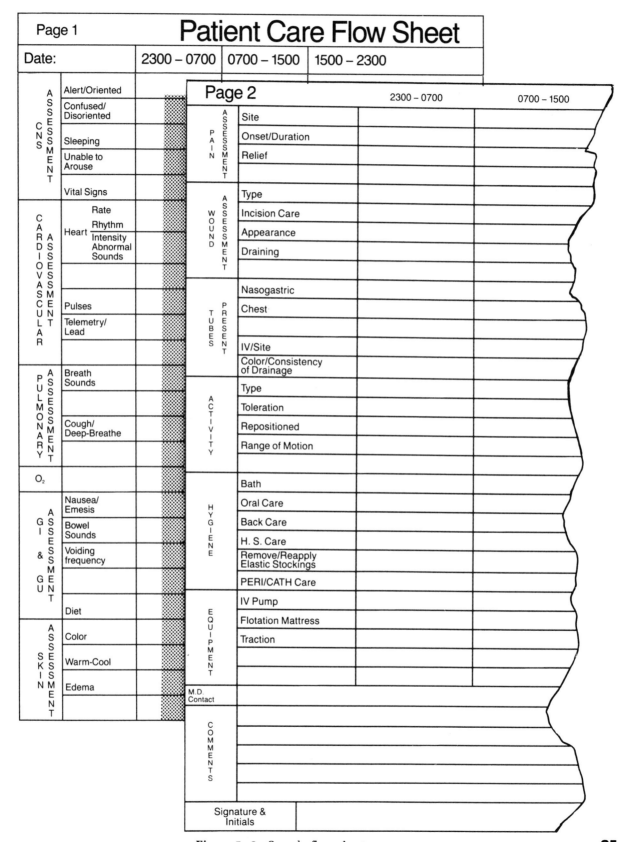

Figure 5-2 Sample flow sheet.

PRACTICE ACTIVITY 5–2

COMMUNICATING NURSING INFORMATION TO OTHER CAREGIVERS

Work through the questions below.

1. Two methods of communicating your observations about patient care and activities to other nurses are by:

   a. _____

   b. _____

2. Discuss the benefits of nursing rounds: _____

   _____

3. Underline the information listed below that you would include in your change-of-shift report:

   Martha ate well   Age 72   Dr. Jefferson
   Weak and unsteady while up in hall   Dressing dry and intact
   3 days postcholecystectomy   Scheduled for discharge tomorrow
   Received oral pain medication at 11 AM with reported relief
   Does not want to go home   Requires instruction in use of walker
   Coordination for home care services in progress with the Discharge Planner

4. The wife of a prominent local politician is admitted for treatment of alcoholism. You could discuss her admission and course of therapy with which of the following people? (check any answers which seem appropriate)

   _____ attending/primary physician

   _____ the nursing supervisor

   _____ a pediatric nurse (her friend)

   _____ your husband

   _____ the patient's son

   _____ an interested newspaper reporter

   _____ other nurses on your unit

dietitian, or physical therapist), the *manner* in which information is conveyed, as well as the content itself, can affect the way in which this information is heard. This, in turn, can impact the quality of the health care provided. For this reason, it is important to avoid judgmental language, tone of voice, or body language. Presenting information in an objective and accurate manner reduces the likelihood of being misunderstood or of negatively influencing the patient's care.

For example: When Martha talked to the nurse, expressing concern about going home, the nurse reported this information to the oncoming shift and to the doctor by saying: "I think Martha is trying to manipulate us. She doesn't want to go home, and she thinks if she 'acts weak,' she won't have to leave the hospital."

After listening to this judgmental report, the oncoming nurse's response might be one of defensiveness and s/he might be inclined to *show* Martha that she is indeed ready to go home. The nurse may also subconsciously stop listening and is likely to be less receptive to what Martha is saying. Contrast the above example with the one which appears below.

> **For example:** If the nurse reports: "Martha has expressed concern about her ability to manage at home. She was weak when we got her up this morning, requiring two people to assist her with walking. We need information about her situation at home and her need for assistance to increase her stamina."

In this report, the nurse expresses a problem in terms that challenge her or him to find a solution. This problem is approached with an open mind, as additional data are gathered and appropriate resources are identified. Maintaining an open mind and actively problem-solving provide opportunities for creating solutions instead of additional problems, thus promoting a positive patient/nurse experience.

The primary format for communicating the patient's current situation and needs is the nursing change-of-shift report. This type of report may be done either in person or via tape recorder. As time for this activity is usually limited, it is necessary to be brief and organized while still providing pertinent data. After supplying basic patient data (e.g., room number, name, age, diagnosis, and physician), reporting may be done "by exception." This means that only occurrences that are out of the ordinary are reported. The nurse notes:

- **Abnormal/changes in assessment findings**
  "Robert developed cyanosis this AM." or "Martha's ankle edema has resolved."
- **Diagnostic procedures and results**
  "Robert's oxygen saturation is 92 percent on 2 liters of oxygen, chest x-ray report is not back yet."
- **Variations from usual routine**
  "Robert was not out of bed this AM but was up for lunch and tolerated it well."
- **Activities not completed on your shift**
  "The walker is in Martha's room, but physical therapy has not been in to instruct her in its use."
- **Status of invasive treatments**
  "Robert's IV of D5 1/2 NS is infusing in the right forearm at 75 ml/hr with 700 ml remaining."
- **Additions or changes to the plan of care** (this includes evaluation of outcomes and the status of patient problems)
  "Robert's Airway Clearance problem has recurred requiring aggressive pulmonary toilet every 2 hours and use of incentive spirometer."

Change-of-shift reports may include *nursing rounds* with each patient being visited by the offgoing and oncoming nurse together. Nursing rounds are beneficial in verifying the status of invasive treatments, appearance of wounds/dressings, and the current condition of the patient (e.g., degree of jaundice, level of coolness of an extremity, etc.). It is imperative to maintain the confidentiality of patient information, and usually it is preferable to review the change-of-shift information before going to the patient's bedside.

Patient confidentiality is an ethical/moral concern that must be respected by each professional at all times. These concerns are extended to conversations at the nursing station, on the telephone, or wherever patient information may be discussed. This includes refraining from discussions with those not directly involved in the patient's care (e.g., staff on other units, your own family, friends, and neighbors).

SUMMARY

In putting the plan of care into action and providing effective patient care, the nurse reviews resources to determine priorities, consulting with and considering the desires of the patient during this Implementation phase of the Nursing Process. The nurse identifies who is responsible for the actions to be taken and what are realistic timeframes. New data are collected in each interaction with the patient and its relevance determined with regard to what is already known. This newly gathered information is documented and shared with other healthcare providers as appropriate. Throughout these activities, flexibility is important to allow for changed circumstances, interruptions, and so forth.

The next chapter will help the nurse to see how continuous evaluation of nursing actions helps to determine whether or not the interventions are leading to successful outcomes. In addition, evaluation of patient plans of care serves as a mechanism for review of the care which is provided on a unit or within an institution. This review process addresses professional issues of overall quality of care and also provides a mechanism by which outside agencies can evaluate the institution.

WORK PAGE: Chapter Five

1. Identify three activities involved in implementing the plan of care:

   a. _____

   b. _____

   c. _____

2. Discuss the importance of understanding the expected effect and potential hazards of the interventions you will implement:

   _____

   _____

   _____

3. Explain the purpose for ongoing data collection throughout the Implementation Phase of the Nursing Process: _____

   _____

   _____

4. List two reasons why documentation of the care provided is important:

   a. _____

   b. _____

5. Name three activities you might use to carry out interventions for planned patient care:

   a. _____   b. _____   c. _____

6. What is the advantage of reporting "by exception"? _____

   _____

7. When and where is patient confidentiality important? _____

   _____

8. Flexibility in providing patient care is important because: _____

   _____

   _____

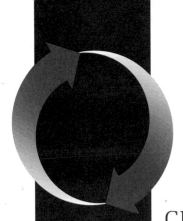

CHAPTER 6

The Evaluation Phase: Determining Whether Desired Outcomes Have Been Met

- Reassessment
- Modification of the Plan of Care
- Termination of Services
- Enhancing Delivery of Quality Care
- Summary

ANA Standard 7: The client's/patient's progress or lack of progress toward goal achievement is determined by the client/patient and the nurse.

ANA Standard 8: The client's/patient's progress or lack of progress toward *goal achievement directs reassessment, reordering of priorities, new goal setting, and revision of the plan of care.*

Evaluation of the patient's response to the care delivered and the achievement of the desired outcomes which were developed in the Planning phase and documented in the plan of care are the final step of the Nursing Process. This evaluation phase is necessary for the determination of how well the plan of care is working, and is an ongoing process. As the patient's condition changes, the patient database changes, requiring revision and updating of the plan of care. The revision of the plan of care is an essential component of the Evaluation phase.

Although the evaluation stage may seem similar to the activity of assessment, there are some important differences. Instead of identifying the patient's general status and problems/needs, the Evaluation phase determines the ap-propriateness of the care provided and the patient's progress or lack of progress toward the desired outcomes. Therefore, evaluation is an interactive, continuous process. As each nursing action is performed, the patient's response is noted and evaluated in relation to the identified outcomes. Then, appropriate actions are taken.

Frequently viewed simplistically as a pass or fail judgment, evaluation should be seen as a constructive opportunity to provide positive feedback to both the patient and caregivers for efforts-to-date, as well as an encouragement to continue to strive for a higher level of functioning or wellness. It is an opportunity for problem-solving and personal growth. The Evaluation phase has three steps: reassessment, modification of the plan of care, and termination of services. The first two steps form a continuous loop of recurring assessment and reaction, which eventually leads to the third step.

REASSESSMENT

Reassessment is an ongoing evaluation process that occurs not just when a desired patient outcome is due to be reviewed or when a determination is needed as to whether or not the patient is ready for discharge. Instead, it is a constant "monitoring" of the patient's status. Data collected as the plan of care was implemented in Step 4 of the nursing process are now evaluated or reassessed. As nursing interventions are accomplished, evaluation of the data collected determines:

- *The appropriateness of the nursing actions*

    For example: Robert's cyanosis has resolved with the provision of oxygen and attention to pulmonary toilet (i.e., periodic deep breathing exercises, effective cough, and position changes).

- *The need to alter the interventions*

    For example: Robert was left in bed for breakfast but should be able to be out of bed for lunch. Or while assisting Martha to walk the length of the hall, you note she is still very weak and unsteady on her feet and will require the assistance of two individuals to provide for patient and employee safety.

- *The development of new patient problems/needs*

    For example: Martha is scheduled for discharge tomorrow. Her current weakness and instability raise concerns about the potential for injury as well as issues of self-care.

- *The need for referral to other resources*

    For example: Martha's physician is notified of your observations, and possible solutions are discussed. Physical therapy may be requested, to provide instruction for Martha in the safe and effective use of a walker. The home health nurse may be contacted to obtain a walker for home use and to supervise Martha's situation postdischarge. Social services may arrange for Meals-on-Wheels to provide a nutritious hot lunch until Martha is able to better care for herself.

- *The need to rearrange priorities to meet the changing demands of care*

    For example: The nurse had planned to get Robert up in the chair for breakfast, but the focused assessment revealed a change in his respiratory status requiring new interventions and revision of the plan. Or the emergency room may call regarding a new patient requiring admission. The nurse needs to review and reschedule the activities planned for Robert and Martha in order to accommodate these additional responsibilities.

While evaluating the patient's response to care, the nurse also notes progress toward the specified outcomes. In addition, as each outcome has an identified timeframe, achievement of the outcomes is periodically reviewed. The nurse must now determine whether the outcomes have been met completely, partially, or not at all; and whether or not the plan of care needs to be revised. Outcome(s) may be evaluated by:

- *Direct observation*

    For example: Did the patient ambulate the length of the hall without developing dyspnea? Did the patient demonstrate proper technique for the administration of insulin? Is the patient free of skin breakdown?

- *Patient interview*

    For example: Does the patient report decreased level of pain following administration of oral medications? Can the patient list resources that are available? Is the patient able to verbalize the signs/symptoms that require medical evaluation or follow-up?

- *Review of records*

    For example: Has the patient's temperature remained within normal range? Are the intake and output balanced? Has the patient gained weight?

An important aspect of this process is the involvement of the patient. How does the patient believe s/he is doing? Discussion of the patient's point of view can provide important insights that will provide additional data for evaluating and revising the plan of care.

If the outcomes were completely met, ask yourself "Which interventions can be terminated"; "How easily were the outcomes achieved"; and "Can timelines be shortened?" To determine *why* an outcome was not met, questions such as those noted in Box 6–1 may help to provide clarification.

BOX 6–1 UNMET OUTCOMES—QUESTIONS TO ASK

If the outcomes have not been met completely, questions to be considered are:

- Were the outcomes realistic and appropriate?
- Was the patient involved in setting the outcomes?
- Does the patient believe the outcomes were important?
- Does the patient know why the outcomes have not been met?
- Have all the interventions that were identified been carried out and in the timeframe specified?
- If not, why not? Were they too vague or misinterpreted?
- What variables may have affected achievement of the outcomes?
- Were new problems/adverse patient responses detected early enough to make appropriate changes in the plan of care?

PRACTICE ACTIVITY 6–1

EVALUATING PATIENT OUTCOMES

Read over the case-study information below. It has been used to develop a plan of care for Mike.

When Mike was admitted to the hospital the evening of 3/11, a physiologic or survival need of pain avoidance was identified (i.e., Pain [acute]). A higher level problem of safety or stimulation was noted (i.e., Physical Mobility, impaired) as was a safety need of protection (i.e., Infection, high risk for).

The following morning during the 8:00 AM assessment, Mike indicated he was successful in obtaining relief of pain following periodic injection of analgesics. Mike also determined that deep breathing exercises and focusing his attention on the scenic picture at the foot of his bed helped to minimize the severity of recurrent muscle spasms in his right leg. In addition, frequent weight shifts using the overhead trapeze and range of motion exercises reduced general aches and joint stiffness.

The nurse noticed that most of Mike's breakfast tray was untouched. Mike reported he was not very hungry but did want fruit juice and other fluids. Following the morning bed bath, the dressings were changed and right leg wound was evaluated. Skin edges were pink and serous drainage was odorless. Pin sites were also cleaned and no signs of inflammation noted. At lunch, Mike's intake was poor and he indicated he was having difficulty chewing and opening his mouth.

During the afternoon assessment at 4:30 PM, Mike's nurse verified that Mike understood and was using infection control techniques of proper handwashing and avoidance of contact with wound and pin sites.

When Mike was set up on the side of the bed before his dinner, he complained of dizziness and sharp pain in his right leg, and he became pale and diaphoretic. He was returned to the supine position and a focused assessment was performed, revealing a blood pressure of 92/60. Within 20 minutes, Mike's color had improved, the dizziness was gone, and the pain relieved with medication.

In reviewing the excerpts from Mike's plan of care, complete the status column denoting whether the outcomes have been met **(m)**, *partially met* **(pm)**, *or not met* **(nm)** *appropriately for the timeframes indicated.*

(Practice Activity continued on page 96)

In addition, the nurse reviews the orders and progress notes of all health-care providers and identifies factors that helped or hindered achievement of outcomes. The findings are then documented on the plan of care and/or progress notes as appropriate and shared with the patient.

MODIFICATION OF THE PLAN OF CARE

When you have completed evaluating the outcomes and the plan of care, it may become apparent that the patient's condition has changed in a direction that was or was not anticipated, and that a change in treatment approach is indicated. The plan of care must be modified to reflect these changes.

As basic physiologic needs (such as air, water, food, and safety) are met, nursing care can progress to higher-level problems (such as those connected to self-esteem). Alternatively, problems related to higher-level needs may be put "on hold," while those associated with newly emerging basic needs are addressed. The nurse may identify or activate additional patient/diagnostic statements, goals, and/or desired outcomes and corresponding interventions. You may recall that we mentioned in an earlier chapter that it is difficult to deal with more than three to five patient problems at one time, and there may simply have been too many of them to address in the initial plan of care.

When the desired outcomes are evaluated and determined to be unmet, the reasons for not meeting them should be identified and documented, and then the outcomes are revised or new outcomes written. When revising patient outcomes, keep in mind that the outcomes may simply need to be restated, or have their timeframes lengthened so that the patient can successfully achieve them.

> **For example:** When Donald was first admitted for acute alcoholism and depression, the initial concerns focused on issues of patient safety/ potential for injury, changes in sensory interpretation, anxiety, and general nutrition. When Donald completed his initial withdrawal from alcohol and his physical condition stabilized, nursing attention became focused on previously identified problems concerning individual coping and role performance.

As the plan of care is modified, remember to address the changing needs of the patient/family and the changes in the patient's health status, environment, and therapeutic regimen. To assist in this process, a patient care conference may be scheduled or a consultation with colleagues or other resource people with special knowledge may be necessary to provide additional input and to problem-solve solutions, as necessary.

TERMINATION OF SERVICES

When desired outcomes have been achieved and the broader goals met, termination of care is planned. The nurse now focuses on how the patient will manage on his or her own. While termination of care may occur when all goals/outcomes are met, it is also possible that some may not have been met. The goals/outcomes that have not been met need to be reviewed, and the reasons why they were not met documented. The discharge plans that began at the time of admission and were periodically updated are finalized and put

(*Text continues on page 98.*)

PRACTICE ACTIVITY 6–1 (*Continued*)

Plan of Care: MIKE

Patient: Mike   Age: 20—03/2/70   Sex: M   Admitted: 03/11/90 5:30pm   Dx: Compound Fx R Tibia/Fibula

DATE	PATIENT DIAGNOSTIC STATEMENT	GOAL	INTERVENTIONS	OUTCOMES	STATUS
3/11/90	Pain [acute], related to movement of bone fragments, soft tissue injury/edema evidenced by verbal complaints, guarding, and muscle tension.	Pain-free or controlled by discharge.	1. Maintain limb rest R leg X24 hr to 5pm 3/12. 2. Elevate lower leg with folded blanket. 3. Apply ice to area as tolerated X48 hr to 5pm 3/13. 4. Place cradle over foot of bed. 5. Document complaints and characteristics of pain. 6. Medicate with Demerol 75 mg and Vistaril 25mg, IM q 4 hr, PRN 7. Demonstrate/encourage use of progressive relaxation techniques, deep breathing exercises, visualization. 8. Provide alternate comfort measures, position change, backrub. 9. Encourage use of diversional activities.	Verbalizes relief of pain within 30 min. of administration of meds. Identifies methods that provide relief by 9a—3/12. Uses relaxation skills to reduce level of pain by 9a—3/12.	

Date	Nursing Diagnosis	Goal	Interventions	Expected Outcomes
3/11/90	Infection, high risk for, related to broken skin, traumatized tissues, invasive procedures.	Free of infection.	1. Monitor temp, V.S., q 4 hr. 2. Aseptic dressing change BID 9a—9p and PRN. 3. Pin care per protocol BID 9a—9p. 4. Routine IV site care daily. 5. Document condition of wound, IV, and pin sites q 4 hr. 6. Review ways patient can reduce risk of infection. 7. Cefoxetin 2 qm IV piggyback q 8 hrs 8a—4p—12m.	Identifies and practices interventions to reduce risk of infection by 5p—3/12. Identifies signs/symptoms requiring medical evaluation by 9a—3/13. Achieves timely wound healing free of purulent drainage by discharge.
3/11/90	Physical Mobility, impaired, related to musculoskeletal impairment and pain, evidenced by reluctance to attempt movement, imposed restrictions.	Ambulates safely with assistive device.	1. Monitor circulation/nerve function R leg q 1 hr X24, then q 4 hr. 2. Support R leg fixator during movement. 3. Support feet with footboard. 4. Encourage use of side rails/overhead trapeze for position change. 5. Demonstrate/assist with ROM exercises to unaffected limbs 2 q hr. 6. Assist out of bed, non-wt. bearing 6p—3/12. 7. Instruct in/monitor use of crutches 3/13.	Participates in activities to maintain muscle strength by 9a—3/12. Increases level of activity by 6p—3/12. Demonstrates techniques/behaviors that enable resumption of activities by 3/13. Maintains position of function R leg, free of foot drop—ongoing.

PRACTICE ACTIVITY 6-2

MODIFICATION OF THE PLAN OF CARE

Based on your evaluation, how would you alter Mike's plan of care from Practice Activity 6-1?

_____

_____

_____

_____

_____

_____

into action. The nurse verifies that the patient/significant other have received written and verbal instructions regarding treatments, medications, and activities to be followed/referred to at home. Signs and symptoms which indicate the need for continued contact with the healthcare providers are reviewed. When necessary, referral/contact phone numbers and other information about resources that may be helpful are given to the patient/family. The nurse determines that contact has been made with appropriate providers for follow-up care, as appropriate (e.g., social worker, home health nurse, or equipment suppliers).

Concerns regarding unmet needs, the need for follow-up monitoring, and progress toward long-term goals after discharge were discussed in Chapter 4. Depending upon how your agency has decided to deal with these issues, you may choose to document your findings and patient instructions in a discharge summary, which also identifies additional activities that the patient and family may do to resolve unmet needs and achieve long-range outcomes/goals. This nursing discharge summary may then be given to the patient. Table 6-1 shows how patient teaching information can be organized and conveyed to the patient.

Even though the patient has been discharged, it is important for the patient and family to know what has been accomplished and what they can continue to do to enhance their own health status in the future. In addition, the discharge summary may be shared with the home care nurse/nurse practitioner and possibly sent to the primary/involved physician for inclusion in the office record. These healthcare providers can promote continued work and monitor progress/changing needs.

Table 6-1 *EXAMPLE OF PATIENT TEACHING INFORMATION FOR PATIENT GOING HOME ON ANTIDYSRHYTHMIC MEDICATION*

Dear Patient:
   This drug has been prescribed for you. This is what you should know about your drug to get the most from your therapy.

1. Antidysrhythmics are taken to regulate your heart rhythm.

2. Antidysrhythmic medications may have to be taken for the rest of your life.

3. Quinidine, procainamide hydrochloride (Pronestyl), propranolol (Inderal), and phenytoin (Dilantin) are taken with meals.

4. Do not take your antidysrhythmics concurrently with [fill in appropriate drugs].

5. Always check with your doctor or pharmacist before taking other drugs because interactions may occur. Drugs known to cause interactions include over-the-counter products for nasal congestion, allergy, pain, or obesity. Drugs of abuse such as marijuana may raise the blood pressure and stimulate heart activity and thus increase abnormal heart rhythm.

6. If you forget to take your antidysrhythmic, do not take the forgotten dose. **Do not** try to catch up by taking 2 doses at the same time. Take the next scheduled dose at the usual time.

7. Do not stop taking your drug unless directed by your doctor.

8. If you have any side effects from your drug, call your doctor. Side effects from taking antidysrhythmics include low blood pressure, lightheadedness, gastrointestinal distress, changes in rate or rhythm of the heart, and often blurred vision. Keep a written record of specific effects that are noted and the time of day that they are noted, such as in the morning upon awaking, with meals, or with activity.

9. Weigh yourself weekly. A gain of 1-2 lb a week may be a sign of increased water. Call your doctor if this occurs.

10. Check your feet and ankles for swelling. If this occurs, notify your doctor.

11. Limit your coffee, tea, or cola drinks, since caffeine may cause an increase in abnormal heart rhythm.

12. Store these drugs in a tight, light-resistant bottle to prevent deterioration.

Source: Mathewson Kuhn, M. Pharmacotherapeutics: A Nursing Process Approach, ed 2. F.A. Davis, Philadelphia, 1990, with permission.

ENHANCING DELIVERY OF QUALITY CARE

Evaluation is an important step for determining the success of the plan of care. In addition, evaluation also allows for review of the nursing process itself. Although you evaluate patient care on an individual basis, unit- or agency-based nursing audit committees focus attention on groups of patients. Comparing overall outcomes and noting the effectiveness of specific interventions is the clinical component of evaluation that can become the basis of research validating the Nursing Process. This external evaluation process is the key for refining standards of care and determining the protocols, policies, and procedures necessary for the provision of quality nursing care in a particular agency.

SUMMARY

The Evaluation phase of the Nursing Process evaluates and reports on the current status of the identified patient problems/needs and is based on the outcomes which were developed in the Planning phase. The evaluation process includes the patient, family, and whoever else is involved in the care of the patient. This process is a positive one, in which the patient's responses to the nursing interventions are evaluated to determine whether or not the desired outcomes were achieved. When the findings are analyzed and it is determined that the outcomes have been met, termination of services is begun and discharge planning is completed. However, if the outcomes have not been met (all or in part), the reassessment process is re-initiated to determine why this is the case. The emergence of new information, the occurrence of unexpected complications, or the choice of the wrong nursing diagnosis should be considered as factors contributing to the failure to achieve a desired patient outcome. At this point, the nursing process is re-initiated, and the plan of care is modified to include the newly identified nursing diagnoses, outcomes, and interventions. This modification, in turn, will be reevaluated at an appropriate time.

The broader application of the evaluation process, to the determination of the overall quality of care delivered at a particular institution, is increasingly used to set standards and to supply information about many facets of the care provided by healthcare agencies. When viewed from a positive standpoint as an opportunity for growth, both individually and for the profession as a whole, the Evaluation phase becomes an important step in the effective delivery of patient care, a process to be valued rather than something to be avoided and/or glossed over quickly.

Documenting the findings of the Evaluation phase, as well as each of the previous steps, is an essential part of the Nursing Process and will be discussed in Chapter 7.

WORK PAGE: Chapter Six

1. What is the difference between assessment and evaluation? _____
   _____
   _____

2. What is the primary purpose of the evaluation process? _____
   _____
   _____

3. The evaluation process provides what three opportunities for the patient and nurse?
   a. _____
   b. _____
   c. _____

4. List the three ways in which patient outcomes may be evaluated, and give an example for each:
   a. _____
   b. _____
   c. _____

5. Since it is advisable to deal with only three to five nursing diagnoses at a time, how are needs
   prioritized? _____
   _____
   _____

6. When is consideration of discharge planning begun? _____
   _____

7.

Vignette: Today is Donald's fifth hospital day. At the start of the shift, you have completed a focused assessment to evaluate progress/changes in status of the identified patient problems. Donald's intake yesterday was approximately 3000 calories, and during rounds, you notice he has eaten all of the food on his breakfast tray. He fills out the next day's menu, neglecting to include any vegetables and selecting only one fruit.

Later, during group, Donald talks about his options for employment and says he knows an employment agency and a business where he can check about possible jobs. He also mentions a

Plan of Care: DONALD

Patient: Donald   Age: 46—2/4/44   Sex: M   Admission: 11/09/90 15:40   Dx: Acute Alcoholism/Depression

DATE	PATIENT DIAGNOSTIC STATEMENT	GOAL	INTERVENTIONS	OUTCOMES	STATUS
11/09/90 Problem 4	Nutrition, altered, less than body requirements related to biologic, psychologic, and economic factors as evidenced by reported inadequate food intake, lack of interest in food, body weight 20% below ideal, and poor muscle tone.	Gains weight appropriately.	1. Weigh every other day (even) 8a. 2. Request evaluation by Dietician 11/11. 3. Discuss individual dietary needs and ways to meet them. 4. Review daily dietary choices on patient's menu. 5. Calculate calorie count daily.	Verbalizes understanding of individual needs by 9a—11/14. Intake meets minimum estimated requirements of 3000 cal/day by 9a—11/14. Identifies ways of meeting nutritional needs within limits of financial resources by 9a—11/15. Weight gain of 2 lb by 8a—11/16. *C. Kraiker, RD*	
11/12 Problem 5	Coping, ineffective, individual related to situational crisis of unemployment, personal vulnerability evidenced by reported inability to cope, use of alcohol, insomnia, and diminished problem-solving.	*Short term:* managing own situation effectively. *Long term:* actively seeking employment and expressing sense of self-worth.	1. Assess level of anxiety and Donald's perception of situation. 2. Note verbal/nonverbal behaviors of anxiety. 3. Look in q 2 hr and PRN. 4. Encourage verbalization, expression of feelings of denial/depression/ anger. 5. Discuss normalcy of these feelings.	Verbalizes awareness of sources of anxiety 10a—11/14. Demonstrates congruency between feelings/ behavior 10a—11/15. Demonstrates initial problem-solving skills 10a—11/15. Identifies options and resources available for assistance 10a—11/16.	

| 11/12 Problem 6 | Role performance related to loss of job evidenced by change in perception of self, change in usual responsibilities, maladaptive coping (i.e., use of alcohol). | Accepting current situation. Establishes plan for future. | 6. Identify current coping mechanisms. 7. Note effectiveness/need for change. 8. Discuss/refer to resources: social worker, alcohol counselor, support group, AA. 1. Discuss perceptions and concerns about current situation (loss of job, hospitalization). 2. Acknowledge reality of grieving process related to loss of job. Assist patient to develop plan for finding employment. 3. Makes own contacts regarding job possibilities and reports results. | Verbalizes realistic perception and acceptance of self in changed role 10a—11/14. Develops realistic plans with 2 strategies for job hunting 10a—11/14. Follows through on plan 10a—11/16. R. Smith RN |

friend who would be willing to help him. He says he is realizing that he is really OK, even though the loss of his job was a devastating event for him following so soon after his divorce. He acknowledges that his feelings of anxiety led to an increase in his drinking. He further says he still has feelings of sadness and occasionally feels a sense of despair but believes he will feel better as he begins to get his life back together again. He seems tentative in accepting his need to be involved in AA, saying he does not know "where they meet, or anyone who attends the meetings."

a. **Evaluation:** Based on the above information, evaluate Donald's progress regarding his problems of Nutrition, altered, less than body requirements; Coping, ineffective; and Role Performance, altered.

_____

_____

_____

b. Modification: How would you change Donald's plan of care? _____

_____

_____

c. How might new concerns regarding the patient affect your discharge plans? _____

_____

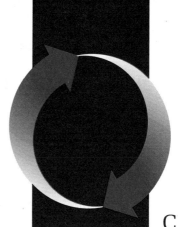

CHAPTER 7

Documenting the Nursing Process

JCAHO Standard MR. 1: The hospital maintains medical records that are documented accurately and in a timely manner, are readily accessible, and permit prompt retrieval of information, including statistical data.

NC. 1.3.5: Nursing care data related to patient assessments, the nursing diagnoses and/or patient needs, nursing interventions, and patient outcomes are permanently integrated into the clinical information system (e.g., the medical record).

ROLE OF DOCUMENTATION

Documentation is not only a requirement for accreditation but is also a legal requirement in *any* healthcare setting. From a nursing focus, documentation provides a record of the use of the nursing process for the delivery of individualized patient care. The initial assessment is recorded in the Patient History or database.

The *identification* of patient problems/needs, and the *planning* of patient care are recorded in the plan of care. The *implementation* of the plan is recorded in the progress notes and/or flow sheets. Finally, the *evaluation* of care may be documented in the progress notes and/or plan of care.

The goals of the documentation system are to:

- Facilitate the quality of patient care.
- Ensure documentation of progress with regard to patient-focused outcomes.
- Facilitate interdisciplinary consistency and the communication of treatment goals and progress.

PROGRESS NOTES

The plan of care that has been developed for a particular patient serves as a framework or outline for the charting of administered care. As noted, this information may be recorded on flow sheets and/or progress notes. Progress notes are an integral component of the overall medical record and should include all significant events which occur in the daily life of the patient. They should be written in a clear and objective fashion and in a manner which reflects progress toward desired measurable outcomes with the use of planned staff interventions. Progress notes have seven major functions as noted in Box 7–1.

Staff Communication

Clearly, staff arriving on the next and subsequent shifts need to know what has been occurring with the patient during the current shift, in order to make appropriate judgments regarding patient management. Colleague-to-colleague communication is the most obvious function of the progress notes, yet this is only a piece of the communication picture. Nursing staff are in the

---

BOX 7–1   SEVEN FUNCTIONS OF PROGRESS NOTES

Progress notes serve multiple functions, and any given note may be written to address one function more than the others. Thus it is important to recognize the seven major functions of progress notes:

1. Staff documentation	5. Training and supervision
2. Legal documentation	6. Reimbursement
3. Evaluation	7. Relationship monitoring
4. Accreditation	

unique position of being in contact with the patient for extended periods of time and in a variety of situations. As a nurse, your observations of patient behavior/response to therapy provide invaluable information to the physician or other provider who may only see the patient for a few minutes each day. Through this communication it can be determined whether the patient's current desired measurable outcomes and interventions need to be eliminated or altered, or if the development of new outcomes or interventions is warranted.

Legal Documentation

In our society, with its many lawsuits and aggressive malpractice emphasis, all aspects of the medical record (including the information contained in daily progress notes) may be important for legal documentation. Progress notes and flow sheets should therefore reflect implementation of the treatment plan as documentation that appropriate actions have been carried out, precautions taken, etc. Both the implementation of interventions and progress toward the measurable outcomes should be documented in the progress notes of the patient's medical record. These notations should also be specific as to date and time and should be signed by the person making the entry. Any errors in the document must be crossed out with one line so that it is still legible, identified by the author as an "error," and then initialed. White-outs or cross-outs which make the information unreadable are not acceptable, as they could be construed to mean that the individual or facility is trying to alter the facts.

Remember, for legal purposes, if an event/activity is not documented, it did not occur or was not done.

Evaluation

Periodic review of the patient's progress and the effectiveness of the treatment plan is completed by the primary nurse and/or the treatment team. An evaluation of the patient's progress may be documented on the plan of care and/or in the progress notes.

For the purpose of reviews (for example, nursing audit committee, state/federal and private agencies such as Board of Health, medicare, JCAHO) the medical record should be written in a manner which facilitates an assessment of the care being given the patient. Progress notes should be written in a manner which reflects work toward the patient's measurable outcomes and the interventions used to attain these outcomes. A person not associated with the healthcare facility should be able to read the notes, determine if the plan of care is being implemented, and also determine whether progress is being made toward measurable outcomes. The medical record should serve as a method of tracking the patient's response to treatment and, consequently, as a means for evaluating the quality of care provided.

Accreditation

The maintenance of a medical record is one of the most essential requirements for healthcare facilities to be accredited by JCAHO and/or other accreditation and licensing agencies. JCAHO standards state that the medical record be documented accurately and in a timely manner. Therefore, the importance of completing notes on schedule and in a manner which facilitates retrieval of

PRACTICE ACTIVITY 7-1

ELEMENTS OF PROGRESS NOTES

Give a brief explanation of how progress notes provide for the following elements of the nurse/patient relationship.

1. *Staff communication:* _____

   _____

2. *Legal documentation:* _____

   _____

3. *Evaluation:* _____

   _____

4. *Accreditation:* _____

   _____

5. *Training:* _____

   _____

6. *Reimbursement:* _____

   _____

7. *Relationship monitoring:* _____

   _____

data should be emphasized. In addition, the new JCAHO standards specify that all patients have a plan of care that is documented in the patient's record.

Training and Supervision

An often underestimated aspect of note writing is the value that such notes hold for training and supervision purposes. An experienced nurse's description of how a complicated situation was handled, a supervisor's analysis of the problems presented by a new admission, and a description of patterns noted in another patient's response to care are all examples of notes which provide models for the remainder of the staff. Supervisors also gain an impression of the employee's abilities through reading progress notes, and may be able to isolate areas in which additional supervision or training/education would be beneficial.

Reimbursement

Third-party reimbursers are insistent that the *why, when, where, how, what,* and *who* of services be clearly documented. An absence of such documentation may result in termination of funding for individual patients and therefore termination of treatment. The medical record is a primary source for maintaining the revenues as well as information about the patient's treatment, providing proof of services. Therefore, progress notes must document any significant observations which show what is happening to the patient during illness, treatment, and recovery. Data about medications, equipment used, and any other pertinent information also need to be recorded.

Relationship Monitoring

The therapeutic relationship which exists between staff and patient is a key factor of treatment in any setting. This **NURSE/PATIENT RELATIONSHIP** is the tool used by the nurse to help the patient make the most of his/her own abilities. In the psychiatric setting, many of the patient's pathologies are manifested in these relationships, and many indications of progress are first identified through the patient's ability to relate more positively and openly with staff as well as peers and family. Thus, monitoring of the patient's relationships is essential, and notes detailing the observed status of these relationships (how the patient interacts in group situations, competitive situations, in one-to-one situations, etc.) have important clinical implications.

NURSE/PATIENT RELATIONSHIP—a therapeutic relationship built on a series of interactions, developing over time, and meeting the needs of the patient.

Finally, regardless of the setting, the patient's relationship with significant other(s) can impact general well-being, progress toward recovery, independence in self-care, and (ultimately) a successful transition to the home setting. Thus, observation and monitoring of these interactions are important components of nursing care.

TECHNIQUES FOR DESCRIPTIVE NOTE-WRITING

Clearly, there is a potentially wide readership for notes written in the medical record that includes coworkers, clinical specialists, physicians, psychiatrists, psychologists, social workers, nurse reviewers, lawyers, judges, utilization reviewers, insurance personnel, surveyors, agency representatives, parents or guardians, as well as the patient. Consideration of this wide readership helps to emphasize the need for clarity and precision in the progress notes.

Since progress notes have many purposes and many potential readers, their clarity and accuracy are essential. From the notes, the reader should be able to form a clear picture of what occurred with the patient. The best way to ensure the clarity of progress notes is through the use of descriptive (or observational) statements. The following is a comparison and contrasting of judgmental language and descriptive language, as well as a guideline for writing observation-based notes.

Judgmental Language

We are all aware of the possibilities for miscommunication which exist in ordinary conversations. The dangers of miscommunication may be even greater when information is conveyed in writing, where the opportunities for clarification which are present in face-to-face communication are absent. We are usually accustomed to speaking and writing in a manner which is judgmental (and therefore ambiguous) without our even being aware of it. Examples of this are noted in Box 7–2. Types of judgmental statements include phrases which:

- Make reference to undefined periods of time
- Refer to undefined quantities
- Refer to qualities
- Fail to specify any objective basis for the judgment made

UNDEFINED PERIODS OF TIME

Statements which refer to undefined periods of time may contain words or phrases such as the following:

often	almost always	most of the time
rarely	frequently	now and then
seldom	occasionally	every so often

Use of these and similar phrases without clarification may leave the statement unclear and judgmental. How often, for example, is "every so often"? Is it every 5 minutes, once an hour, or three times per shift? This is not to say that the staff member must time each and every interaction or occurrence. Rather, one should be aware of the *potential* for confusion in these words. Ask yourself: Does this note concern an event about which a more specific time relationship should be noted? If documenting for potential legal purposes (an injury, for example), specificity will be essential. However, for routine communication purposes, this may not be the case. For example, if

---

BOX 7–2 EXAMPLES OF JUDGMENTAL LANGUAGE

Consider the following statements:

"He asks for pain medication **too often**."
"He is **uncooperative** today."
"She did a **good job** on her incentive spirometer today."
"He is a **manipulative** patient."
"The new patient is really **difficult**."
"He has a **poor** outlook."
"She had a **bad attitude** about doing her physical therapy this morning."

The highlighted words in each of the above statements represent judgments (or conclusions), not facts. Without any elaboration or basis for comparison, each of the statements is a statement of opinion, open to varying interpretations. Contrast these with the statements in Box 7–3.

you note "The patient was quiet for most of the shift today," the exact number of minutes during which she was quiet or not quiet is not necessary for reasonably accurate communication to occur.

UNDEFINED QUANTITIES

Statements which refer to undefined quantities may use such words or phrases as the following:

some	enough	a great deal	too much
a lot	many	very little	large amount

As with the previous statements, each of these terms is open to interpretation. "A lot" of complaints to one person, for example, might mean five; to another it might mean twenty. Or, "a large amount of bloody drainage" could be 200 ml or only 50 ml of fluid. It is generally advisable to avoid undefined quantities.

QUALITIES

All descriptive adjectives applied to patients have the potential to fall under this category, since they may involve making subjective definitions beforehand. Of most concern, however, are words which could be called "semitechnical" in nature:

passive	irritating	incompetent
nervous	manipulative	overprotective
demanding	alcoholic	disturbed

Words such as those above may have connotations in the health field beyond the scope of their ordinary definitions. Therefore, elaboration upon these qualities may be desirable. More common adjectives may have a generally accepted meaning and, therefore, pose less of a problem, and may have less potential for misunderstanding. However, observed behaviors may call for conclusions on your part which are influenced by your own biases and cultural background. It is best to check out these understandings with others and particularly with the patient before using the following types of terms:

friendly	unhappy	enthusiastic	proud
attentive	excited	bored	observant
aloof	apathetic	cheerful	happy

Finally, there are slang words (used informally), which besides being unclear because they are used only by small subcultural groups, should not be contained in a professionally written note in any case:

hyped-up	spaced-out	bummed	crazy
loose	pushy	cool	tanked-up

OBJECTIVE BASIS FOR JUDGMENTS

Some statements are self-evidently a judgment on the part of the observer and are offered without any objective basis. Such statements may cause the reader to ask, "How do you **know** that this patient . . ."

- is improving?

BOX 7–3 PROVIDING AN OBJECTIVE BASIS FOR YOUR JUDGMENTS

Consider the following statements. Although the highlighted words represent a judgment or conclusion, objective facts or behavioral observations are provided to support or substantiate the judgment.

Mike **is improving**; he walked the length of the hall using his crutches.

Robert **has a good attitude**, expressing optimism that he will be able to prevent a recurrence of pneumonia.

Martha **enjoys reading**, spending 3–4 hours a day in this activity.

Donald **expresses anger** toward his roommates' smoking, loud conversations with visitors, and commandeering of the TV. (*Note:* Making the inference that Donald **hates his roommate** from his expression of anger results in an unclear or unsupported judgment.)

- has a good attitude?
- enjoys reading?
- hates his roommate?

Recording your observations and providing an objective basis for your judgments (as in Box 7–3) will reduce the possibility of miscommunication or misinterpretation, and the reader will not have to look elsewhere for clarification.

Descriptive Language

As noted above, descriptive language contains observations only and avoids statements which are evaluative or judgmental unless observational evidence can be presented to back up the judgment. You will remember that being able to actually observe the patient doing something was the criterion of a well-written outcome. The situation is similar for observation-based progress notes; properly written objective statements refer to specific observable or measurable events. Descriptive statements:

- *Contain measurable periods of time*

   For example:

ten times in 1 hour	every half hour	15 minutes
once	48 hours	four times a day

- *Contain measurable quantities*

   For example:

twenty percent of the diet	all of the patients
six out of eight	completely saturated
none	5 ml

- *Provide a basis or rationale for qualities named in the note*

   For example:

   1. Sally is nervously awaiting the physician's visit, twisting a

handkerchief and repeatedly questioning whether the doctor has arrived.

  2. Jennifer's mother is demanding, repeatedly asking for immediate nursing attention for minor needs.
  3. Donald is passive, responding to the nurse's questions regarding scheduling of his care by replying "whatever you want to do."

You may have gotten the impression in the preceding section that you can never use adjectives in your notes. This is far from the case. In fact, you *should* give your impressions of the patient.

Statements in which you note that the patient "seemed" or "appeared" to be exhibiting a certain physical/emotional state are inferential statements. These are a subset of descriptive statements in which you infer the patient's state based on your observations of their behavior and interactions, your knowledge of the patient's patterns, and the connections you make between behavior/affect and what has been happening during the illness. Such statements are often of great value.

However, you should not allow your subjective impressions to stand alone, particularly if your observation involves some of the more "semitechnical" qualities noted earlier. You should also provide some reasons why you believed the patient was "improving," "demanding," "manipulative," or whatever.

For example:

  1. "Robert seemed upset by the news, as evidenced by the fact that he turned on his side and would not speak to caregivers."
  2. "Consistent with the pattern noted previously, Donald reacted to the change in his treatment plan by becoming upset and angry."
  3. "Martha appeared to be frustrated, verbally expressing her dismay at her inability to walk around the room unassisted."

When comparisons or judgments *are* made, a descriptive statement should state the source or basis of judgment.

For example:

  1. Based on the patient's laboratory reports . . .
  2. Psychologic testing showed that . . .
  3. The other patient stated that . . .
  4. Judging by the fact that . . .

Also note that whenever the source of a judgment is specified, the statement becomes a behavioral report. Because such a report can be observed, this type of statement is an observation and is therefore descriptive. Consider the differences between the following two statements.

For example:

  1. The patient is weaker today.
  2. Physical therapy reports, "Martha is weaker today."

The first statement is clearly judgmental because of the undefined phrase "weaker today." The second, however, is an observable event. Obviously (although physical therapy may be wrong), it is an objective fact that the physical therapist said that the patient is weaker today. It may help to think of such statements as quotations. *What* the physical therapist said does not influence our ability to observe him or her saying it, and then objectively reporting that observation.

Finally, the nurse can chart observations in a nonjudgmental manner. "Martha displayed increased weakness, was unsteady on her feet, and required the assistance of two persons to maintain balance." In Box 7–4, additional examples further illustrate how judgmental statements may be interpreted and restated more objectively.

Content of Note/Entry

The term "progress note" indicates that the patient's *progress* is to be documented along with the implementation of the treatment plan. Contents should be as specific and exact as possible.

For communication purposes it is important to record in the progress notes any information which is of importance to oncoming shifts as well as

---

BOX 7–4 COMPARISON OF JUDGMENTAL AND BEHAVIORAL NOTES

The important thing to know about judgmental statements is that they can be translated into more precise terms. For example:

Judgmental: "The patient did pretty well today."
Behavioral: "The patient followed directions for drawing up and administering her insulin without any mistakes."

Judgmental: The meeting with the physical therapist did not go very well.
Behavioral: The patient stated she "could not do the exercises which were to be started today."

Judgmental: The patient had a bad attitude all day.
Behavioral: The patient argued with staff five times during the shift.

Judgmental: The patient became aggressive.
Behavioral: The patient clenched his fists and yelled to the nurse, "I'd like to hit you." He then hit the wall twice with his fist.

Judgmental: The patient would not follow directions.
Behavioral: The patient drank a glass of water 30 minutes before his scheduled surgery in spite of reminders to remain NPO.

Judgmental: The patient ate poorly.
Behavioral: Patient ate ⅓ of her lunch (all of the broccoli and corn, no meat, potatoes, or bread) and drank 50 mL of apple juice.

As you can see from the above examples, it often takes a bit more thought to write a note which is objectively descriptive. However, the benefits in clarity of communication make the effort essential for the many purposes of progress notes.

observations you have made which may be significant for other healthcare providers. Box 7–5 profiles what information should be included. Remember, you are actually charting for the future. You know what is happening today. However, the reader of tomorrow, next week, or next year must rely on your written words in order to share your understanding of the patient's situation at a given moment.

Thus, when applying restraints, for example (which constitutes a "major event with both therapeutic and legal ramifications"), the exact time the procedure was initiated, whether any injuries resulted, and so on should be documented. It is also necessary to document what led up to the situation, how staff and other participants reacted, what less restrictive measures were tried, and any significant observations regarding the incident. An example of how to document a therapeutic event is presented in Box 7–6.

Other areas of concern which enhance accurate communication are the use of correct grammar and spelling, legible writing, and the use of nonerasable ink. Avoiding the repetition of data when possible promotes clarity of documentation. Since this is "the patient's record," it is not necessary to use the term "the patient"; however, periodically using the patient's name can avoid problems if parts of the record become separated. Having a name noted can help to identify the proper chart and prevent problems of charting on the wrong record. Abbreviations should be used with caution or avoided in most instances. Although some institutions provide a list of approved abbreviations which identifies the correct meanings, abbreviations can be misleading or easily misinterpreted, resulting in misunderstandings and errors with serious consequences. For example, a patient reading his record might not realize that "SOB" stands for short of breath.

Last, but *not* least, remember to be brief. Entries need to be concise, short, succinct sentences or phrases that provide enough information to communicate your observations, thoughts, and plans. The entry needs to be consistent in style and format to avoid confusion and to comply with agency policies. Avoid repetition/redundancy. Do not rewrite what is already recorded on flow sheets but do use the progress note to expand on the flow sheet and to note the patient's response. For example: when documenting your repeat assessment of a wound, you may chart "no change" if your baseline observations are previously recorded.

Format of Note/Entry

There are several charting formats that have been used for documentation. These include: block notes, with a single entry covering an entire shift (e.g., 7–3 PM); narrative timed notes (e.g., 8:30 AM, Ate all of breakfast); and the problem-oriented medical record system (**POMR** or **PORS**) using the **SOAP/SOAPIER** approach (Box 7–7), to name a few. The latter can provide thorough documentation, but it was designed by physicians for episodic care and requires that the entries be tied to a patient problem identified from a problem list.

A new system format created by nurses for documentation of frequent/repetitive care is FOCUS® Charting. It was designed to encourage looking at the patient from a positive rather than a negative (or problem-oriented) perspective by using precise documentation to record the nursing process. Recording

POMR OR PORS—Problem-Oriented Medical Record—a method of recording data about the health status of the patient.

SOAP—format for documentation—subjective, objective, analysis, plan.

WRITING NONJUDGMENTAL STATEMENTS

*Identify the statements that are judgmental (**J**) and those that are observational/behavioral (**O/B**).*
Rewrite the judgmental notes to reflect behavioral language:

1. Mrs. Jewel has a poor body image since undergoing a mastectomy. _____

   _____

2. Mr. Dunn needs to be evaluated regarding his competence to manage his household affairs since his stroke. _____

   _____

3. Miss Janus usually practices breast self-examination. _____

   _____

4. Mary Bird does not eat enough for her current level of activity. _____

   _____

5. Mrs. Lambert stops taking her medication; then when she has a seizure, she presents at the doctor's office for treatment. _____

   _____

6. It has been a long time since Mr. Babbit has had his medications evaluated. _____

   _____

BOX 7-5 CONTENT OF SUCCESSFUL PROGRESS NOTES

Examples of the kind of information which is important to record in the progress notes include:

- *Unsettled or unclear problems or "issues"* which need to be dealt with, including attempts to contact other healthcare providers
- *Noteworthy incidents or interviews* involving the patient that would benefit from a more detailed recording
- *Other pertinent data* such as notes on phone calls, home visits, and family interactions
- *Additional critical incident data* such as seemingly significant or revealing statements made by the patient, an insight you have into a patient's patterns of behavior, patient injuries, the use of any special treatment procedure, or other major events such as episodes of pain, respiratory distress, panic attacks, medication reactions, suicidal comments
- *Administered care, activities, or observations* if not recorded elsewhere on flow sheets (physician visits, completion of ordered tests, nonroutine medications, etc.)

BOX 7–6   DOCUMENTING A THERAPEUTIC EVENT

Thirty-six hours after Donald was admitted to the unit with a diagnosis of acute alcoholism, he became disoriented to time/place and person, was extremely agitated, and was "picking in the air" saying he was trying to "catch the bugs." He was given medication and placed in restraints in a seclusion room with the door open. This was charted as follows:

4:00 PM: Became agitated without notice. Medicated with librium, reoriented to place/events in quiet tones as staff paced with him, and reinforced that he would be kept safe. Agitation escalated, unable to remain in one place for any significant period of time, expressed fear of the "things" he was seeing. Agreed to use of restraints to help keep him safe until he could regain control and/or medication became effective.

4:15 PM: Procedure explained as Donald was put in seclusion room C and placed in 4-point wrist/ankle restraints without incident or injury. Informed that door would remain open and a staff member would check on him every 10 minutes or more frequently as needed. Vital signs: B/P 150/90, Pulse 120, Respirations 28.

4:20 PM: Dr. Carter notified of current status.

BOX 7–7   COMPONENTS OF THE SOAP/SOAPIER CHARTING FORMAT

The **SOAP** format is generally used for the initial assessment of the patient. Once the plan of care is implemented and the evaluation process begun, the **SOAPIER** format becomes more appropriate.

Subjective: statements from patient/others
Objective: measurable or observable data
Analysis: interpretations/conclusions based on the above information
Plan: what is to be done about the identified problem(s)
Implementation: what or how plan is carried out
Evaluation: patient's response to the interventions
Revision: how the plan of care will be changed

BOX 7–8 COMPONENTS OF THE FOCUS® CHARTING FORMAT

Focus: Nursing diagnosis, patient problem/concern, sign/symptom, event

Data: Subjective/objective information describing and/or supporting the focus

Action: Immediate/future nursing actions based on assessment and consistent with/complementary to the goals and nursing action recorded in the patient plan of care

Response: Describes the effects of interventions and whether or/not the goal/outcome was met

of assessment, interventions, and evaluation information in a DAR (Data, Action, and Response) format (Box 7–8) facilitates tracking and following what is happening to the patient at any given moment. Charting focuses on patient and nursing concerns. The focal point is patient status and the associated nursing care. The Focus is always stated in a way that reflects the *patient's* concern/need rather than reflecting a nursing task or medical diagnosis. Box 7–9 highlights some of the distinguishing features of a Focus.

BOX 7–9   WHAT IS A FOCUS?

The nurse often speaks of "a focus" for her assessment, diagnosis, and planning of care.

- A patient problem/concern or nursing diagnosis,

     For example:

     Airway   Nutrition
     Fluid Excess   Knowledge Deficit, wound care

     The "stem" or diagnostic label is taken from the plan of care. You do not need to waste time and space in repeating the entire diagnostic statement.

- Signs/symptoms of potential importance

     For example:

     fever   dysrhythmia
     nausea   hypotension
     confusion   edema

     These require monitoring or limited intervention, but if the signs and symptoms persist, a patient problem will be identified and added to the plan of care.

     For example:
     continued nausea can affect fluid volume; dysrhythmias and hypotension may develop into a cardiac output concern.

- Significant event or change in status
     For example:

     admission/transfer   seizure
     fall out of bed   respiratory arrest

     A single incident may evolve into a patient problem for inclusion in the plan of care.

     For example: a fall raises concerns about High Risk Injury or possibly, Thought Processes, altered, if confusion is present; or a respiratory arrest may be related to Airway Clearance or Breathing Pattern, ineffective.

- Specific standards of care/hospital policy
     For example:

     admission/discharge summary   preoperative visit
     routine shift assessment   discharge planning

Whatever documentation system you use, an organized format is a method of identifying, working through, and solving the patient's problems. SOAP and FOCUS® notes help to organize your thinking and provide structure within which creative problem-solving is more likely to occur. Structured communication promotes consistency between various services/healthcare providers. Compare the charts in Tables 7–1 and 7–2 for Richard, an NIDDM patient, with ulceration of the left foot.

SOAPIER—format for documentation— subjective, objective, analysis, plan, implementation, evaluation, revision.

SUMMARY

The use of clear documentation techniques for planning, implementing, and evaluating patient care helps the nurse to effectively individualize patient care, set priorities, and provide a picture of what *has* happened and what *is* happening to promote continuity of care as well as ongoing evaluation. This, in turn, reinforces each individual nurse's accountability and responsibility for using the nursing process. As documentation skills are improved, time will be saved by the consistent use of a documentation system which focuses on specific issues. This documentation of professional nursing care can also help in meeting legal and accreditation requirements, without an additional expenditure of valuable time in information gathering.

Table 7–1 SAMPLE SOAP/SOAPIER CHARTING FORMAT FOR RICHARD

DATE	TIME	NUMBER/PROBLEM*	SOAP/SOAPIER FORMAT†
6/30/91	1400	#1 (Skin Integrity)	**S:** "That hurts" (when tissue surrounding wound is palpated). **O:** Scant amount serous drainage on dressing. Wound borders pink. No odor present. **A:** Wound shows early signs of healing, free of infection. **P:** To continue skin care per care plan. In order to document more of the nursing process, some institutions have added the following: Implementation, Evaluation, Revision (if plan was ineffective) **I:** Betadine soaks as ordered. Applied sterile dressing with paper tape. **E:** Wound clean, no drainage present. Signed: *E. Moore RN*
6/28/91	2100	#2 (Pain)	**S:** Complains of "dull, throbbing pain in left foot," states there is no radiation to other areas. **O:** Muscles tense. **A:** Persistent pain. **P:** Foot cradle placed on bed. Darvon 65 mg given po. Signed: *M. Seabrook RN*
	2130		**E:** Reports pain relieved. Appears relaxed. Signed: *B. Marsh RN* *(Continued)*

Table 7-1   SAMPLE SOAP/SOAPIER CHARTING FORMAT FOR RICHARD (*Continued*)

DATE	TIME	NUMBER/PROBLEM*	SOAP/SOAPIER FORMAT†
6/30/91	1100	#3 (Knowledge Deficit, diabetic teaching)	**S:** Listed questions/concerns of self and wife. (Copy attached to teaching plan.) **O:** None **A:** Richard and wife need review of information and practice for insulin administration. **P:** Attend group teaching session with wife and meet with dietitian. Read "Understanding Your Diabetes." **I:** He demonstrated insulin administration technique for wife to observe. Provided procedure handout sheet for future reference. Scheduled meeting for them with dietitian at 1300 today to discuss remaining questions. **E:** Richard more confident in demonstration, performed activity without hesitation, correctly and without hand tremors. Richard explained steps of procedure and reasons for actions to wife. Couple identified resources to contact if questions/problems arise. Signed: *E. Moore RN*

* As noted on Plan of Care.
†**S** = Subjective: statements from patients/others
  O = Objective: measurable or observable data
  A = Analysis: interpretations/conclusions based on the above information
  P = Plan: what is to be done about the identified problem(s)

Table 7-2   SAMPLE OF FOCUS® CHARTING FOR RICHARD

DATE	TIME	FOCUS*	FOCUS: DAR FORMAT
6/30/91	1400	Skin Integrity, L foot	**D:** Scant amount serous drainage on dressing, wound borders pink, no odor present, denies discomfort except with direct palpation of surrounding tissue. **A:** Betadine soak as ordered. Sterile dressing applied with paper tape. **R:** Wound clean—no drainage present. Signed: *E Moore RN*
6/28/91	2100	Pain, L foot	**D:** Complaining of dull/throbbing ache L foot—no radiation. Muscles tense. **A:** Foot cradle placed on bed. Darvon 65 mg given po. Signed: *M. Suhr RN*
	2200	Pain, L foot	**R:** Reports pain relieved. Appears relaxed. Signed: *B Marsh RN*

(*Continued*)

Table 7–2   SAMPLE OF FOCUS® CHARTING FOR RICHARD (*Continued*)

DATE	TIME	FOCUS*	FOCUS: DAR FORMAT
6/30/91	1100	Knowledge Deficit, diabetic teaching	**D:** Attended group teaching session with wife. Both have read "Understanding Your Diabetes." **A:** Reviewed list of questions/concerns from Richard and wife. (Copy attached to teaching plan.) Richard demonstrated insulin administration technique for wife to observe. Provided procedure handout sheet for future reference. Scheduled meeting for them with dietitian at 1300 today to discuss remaining questions. **R:** Richard more confident in demonstration, performed activity without hesitation, correctly and without hand tremors. He explained steps of procedure and reasons for actions to wife. Couple identified resources to contact if questions/problems arise. Signed: *E Moore RN*

The following is an example of documentation of a patient need/concern that currently does not require identification as a patient problem (nursing diagnosis) or inclusion in the plan of care and therefore not easily documented in the SOAP format:

6/29/87	2020	Gastric distress	**D:** Awakened, complains of "indigestion/burning sensation" with hand over epigastric area. Skin warm/dry, color pink, vital signs unchanged. **A:** Given Mylanta 30 ml po. Head of bed elevated approximately 15 degrees. **R:** Reports pain relieved. Appears relaxed, resting quietly. *E Moore RN*

* **D** = Data
 A = Action
 R = Response

Source: FOCUS® Charting, Susan Lampe, RN, MS, "Creative Nursing Management, Inc.," 614 East Grant Street, Minneapolis, MN 55404.

WORK PAGE: Chapter Seven

1. You are to present information regarding documentation. Identify three goals of the documentation process you will include in your presentation:

a. _____

b. _____

c. _____

2. Steps of the Nursing Process are documented on which form:

a. Plan of care   _____ Assessment

b. Progress notes   _____ Problem identification

c. Patient database   _____ Planning

d. Flow sheets   _____ Implementation

                         _____ Evaluation

3. List five functions of progress notes:

a. _____

b. _____

c. _____

d. _____

e. _____

4. JCAHO standards mandate that the medical record shall contain the following elements of nursing care data:

a. _____

b. _____

c. _____

d. _____

5. In documenting for reimbursement, five factors need to be included: These are: _____

_____

_____

6. Two ways in which the plan of care can be used for supervision are: _____

_____

7. The best way to ensure clarity of the progress notes is: _____

_____

_____

8. Rewrite the following judgmental statements to make them more nonjudgmental:

   a. He is uncooperative today.

_____

   b. He is a manipulative patient.

_____

   c. She had a bad attitude about taking her medication this morning.

_____

   d. The new patient is really difficult.

_____

9. List three types of judgmental statements:

   a. _____

   b. _____

   c. _____

10. Name three types of data which are important to record in the progress notes:

   a. _____

   b. _____

   c. _____

11. List five additional factors which can enhance accurate communication: _____

_____

_____

12. What actions can be taken to correct an error in charting? _____

_____

13. Name three charting formats: _____

_____

14. Read the following Vignette and record the patient data using the SOAP format, the FOCUS format, and the format used in your institution, if different:

Vignette: Sally is admitted to your unit in active labor at 38 weeks gestation. As you oriented Sally to her surroundings, you began the assessment process. Sally has taken childbirth classes with her husband, who is currently returning from a business trip to a nearby city. Her mother is at home with Sally's children. Strong contractions are now 4 to 5 minutes apart and last 40 seconds. Cervix is dilated to 5 cm. Sally is complaining of constant low backache and is moving about restlessly in the bed, unable to find a comfortable position. She asks you to contact her physician—"I need medication for pain now." (Sally's physician is presently attending a birth in another local hospital.) You note she is not using breathing or relaxation techniques. She becomes teary-eyed with contractions and repeats, "What's taking my husband so long to get here!" Your first response is to help Sally regain control of the situation and reduce her level of pain. You reposition pillows to provide better support, quickly straighten bed linens, talk about the distance her husband is traveling, and reinforce anticipated travel time, while administering a backrub. As the next contraction begins, you encourage Sally to use learned breathing techniques while you continue to massage her back. Afterward, you suggest Sally call home and speak with her mother. You tell Sally that someone will remain with her as she needs. As the next contraction begins, Sally is able to focus her attention appropriately and use learned behaviors to maintain control. When the contraction passes, you note Sally appears comfortably relaxed and says she wishes to rest and will call when she needs something. As you leave the room, you inform Sally that you will return within 15 minutes if she does not need you sooner.

COMPREHENSIVE WORK SHEET

PUTTING TOGETHER WHAT YOU HAVE LEARNED ABOUT THE NURSING PROCESS

Review the following vignette and nursing history. Then, create a plan of care for your patient, Mr. Simmons. Identify two patient problems/needs, writing the patient diagnostic statement and two outcomes. Choose three interventions for each problem/need.

Vignette: Mr. A. Simmons, noninsulin-dependent diabetic (NIDDM) for 5 years, presented to his physician's office with a nonhealing ulcer of 3 weeks' duration, on his left foot. Lab studies at that time revealed blood sugar of 256 per finger stick and urine clinitest of 1%/small.

Admitting Physician's Orders

Culture/Sensitivity and gram stain of foot ulcer
Random blood sugar on admission and fingerstick BG every AM
CBC, electrolytes, glycosylated Hb in AM
Chest x-ray & ECG in AM
NPH insulin 15u q AM. Begin insulin instruction for self care post discharge
Dicloxacillin 500 mg po, q 6 h, start after culture obtained
Darvon 65 mg q 4 h prn, pain
Diet—2400 cal ADA/3 meals with 2 snacks
Up in chair ad lib with feet elevated
Foot cradle for bed
Betadine soak L foot tid × 15 min, then cover with dry sterile dressing
Vital signs q.i.d.

Patient Assessment Database

Name: R. Simmons   **Informant:** Patient   **Reliability (Scale 1–4):** 3
Age: 64   **DOB:** 5/3/27   **Race:** Caucasian   **Sex:** M
Adm. date: 6/28/91   **Time:** 7 PM   **From:** Home

ACTIVITY/REST

Reports (Subjective)

Occupation: Farmer
Usual activities/hobbies: reading, playing cards. "Don't have time to do much. Anyway I'm too tired most of the time to do anything after the chores."
Limitations imposed by illness: "have to watch what I order if I eat out."
Sleep: Hours: 6–8 hrs/night   **Naps:** No   **Aids:** No
Insomnia: "Not unless I drink coffee after supper."
Usually feels rested when awakens at 4:30 AM.

Exhibits (Objective)

Observed response to activity: favors L foot when walking
Mental status: Alert/active

Neuro/muscular assessment: muscle mass/tone: bilaterally equal/firm
   Posture: erect   **ROM:** full
   Strength: equal 3 extremities/favors L foot currently

CIRCULATION

Reports (Subjective)

History of slow healing: lesion L foot, 3 weeks.
Extremities: Numbness/Tingling: "my feet feel cold and tingling when I walk a lot."
Cough/character of sputum: occ./white.
Change in frequency/amount of urine: yes, voiding more lately.

Exhibits (Objective)

Peripheral pulses: Radials 3+, popliteal, dorsalis, post tibial, pedal, all 1+.
B/P: R: Sit: 140/86   **Lying:** 146/90   **Stand:** 138/90
       L: Sit: 138/88   **Lying:** 142/88   **Stand:** 138/84
Pulse: Apical: 86   **Radial:** 86   **Quality:** strong   **Rhythm:** regular
Chest auscultation: few rhonchi clear with cough, no murmurs/rubs
Jugular vein distention: –0–
Extremities:
  Temperature: Feet cool bilat/remainder warm.
  Color: skin: legs pale
  Capillary refill: slow both feet
  Homan's sign: –0–   **Varicosities:** few enlarged superficial veins both calves
  Nails: Toenails thickened, yellow, brittle
  Distribution and quality of hair: coarse hair to midcalf, none on toes
Color: General: ruddy face/arms   **Mucous membranes/lips:** pink
  Nail beds: blanch well   **Conjunctiva and sclera:** white

EGO INTEGRITY

Reports (Subjective)

Report of stress factors: "Normal farmer's problems: weather, pests, bankers, etc."
Ways of handling stress: "I get busy with the chores and talk things over with my livestock, they
   listen pretty good."
Financial concerns: No insurance/needs to hire someone while here.
Relationship status: married   **Cultural factors:** rural/agrarian
Religion: Protestant/practicing
Lifestyle: middle class/self sufficient farmer   **Recent changes:** no
Feelings: "I'm in control of most things, except this diabetes now."

Exhibits (Objective)

Emotional status: Calm
Other: concerned re possible therapy change "from pills to shots"
Observed physiologic response(s): occasionally sighs deeply/frowns, shrugs shoulders

ELIMINATION

Reports (Subjective)

Usual bowel pattern: most every PM
Last BM: last night   **Character of stool:** firm/brown
Bleeding: –0–   **Hemorrhoids:** –0–   **Constipation:** occ.

Laxative used: Hot prune juice.
Urinary: no problems   **Character of urine:** pale yellow

Exhibits (Objective)

Abd. tender: No   **Soft/Firm:** soft   **Palpable mass:** None
Bowel sounds: active all 4 quads.

FOOD/FLUID

Reports (Subjective)

Usual diet (type): 2400 ADA (occ. "cheats" with dessert, "but my wife watches it pretty closely.")   **# meals daily:** 3/1 snack
Dietary Pattern: B: fruit juice/toast/ham/coffee
              L: meat/potatoes/veg/fruit/milk
              D: meat sandwich/soup/fruit/coffee
Snack: milk/crackers at HS.   **Usual beverage:** skim milk, 2–3 cups decaf coffee, and drinks *lots* of water.
Last meal/intake: Dinner: roast beef sandwich, vegetable soup, pear with cheese, decaf
Loss of appetite: "Never, but lately I don't feel as hungry as usual."
Nausea/Vomiting: –0–   **Food Allergies:** none
Heartburn/food intolerance: cabbage causes gas
Mastication/swallowing probs: No   **Dentures:** partial upper plate
Usual weight: 175   **Recent changes:** has lost about 3# this month.
Diuretic therapy: No

Exhibits (Objective)

Wt: 171#   **Ht:** 5'10"   **Build:** stocky   **Skin turgor:** good/leathery
Appearance of tongue: midline, pink   **mucous membranes:** pink, intact
Condition of teeth/gums: good, "no problem with bleeding."
Breath sounds: few rhonchi cleared with cough.
Bowel sounds: active all 4 quads
Urine Chemstix: 1%/small

HYGIENE

Reports (Subjective)

Activities of Daily Living: Independent in all areas.
Preferred time of bath: PM

Exhibits (Objective)

General appearance: clean, shaven, short cut hair. Hands rough and dry.
Scalp & eyebrows: scaly white patches

NEUROSENSORY

Reports (Subjective)

Headache: "occasionally behind my eyes when I worry too much"
Tingling/Numbness: my feet, occasionally
Eyes: vision loss, far-sighted   **Exam:** 2 yrs. ago.
Ears: Hearing loss   **R:** "some"   **L:** No (has not been tested)
Nose: Epistaxis: –0–   **Sense of smell:** states no problem.

Exhibits (Objective)

Mental status: alert, oriented to time, place, person.
 Affect: concerned   **Memory: Remote/Recent:** clear and intact
Speech: clear/coherent
Pupil reaction: PERLA   **Glasses:** Reading   **Hearing Aid:** No
Handgrip/release: strong/equal

PAIN/DISCOMFORT

Reports (Subjective)

Location: L foot   **Intensity (1–10):** 5 to 6   **Quality:** dull ache
Frequency/Duration: "seems like all the time"   **Radiation:** no
Precipitating factors: shoes, walking   **How relieved:** ASA, not helping
Other complaints: sometimes has back pain following chores/heavy lifting relieved by ASA/linament rubdown.

Exhibits (Objective)

Facial grimacing: when lesion border palpated.
Guarding affected area: pulls foot away.   **Narrowed focus:** No
Emotional response: tense, irritated.

RESPIRATION

Reports (Subjective)

Dyspnea: –0–   **Cough:** Occ. morning cough, white sputum.
Emphysema: –0–   **Bronchitis:** –0–   **Asthma:** –0–   **Tuberculosis:** –0–
Smoker: Filters   **pk/day:** ½   **# of years:** 40+
Use of respiratory aids: –0–

Exhibits (Objective)

Respiratory rate: 22   **Depth:** good   **Symmetry:** equal, bilateral
Auscultation: few rhonchi, clear with cough.
Cyanosis: –0–   **Clubbing of fingers:** –0–
Sputum characteristics: none to observe.
Mentation/restlessness: alert/oriented/relaxed

SAFETY

Reports (Subjective)

Allergies: –0–   **Blood transfusions:** –0–
Sexually Transmitted Disease: None
Fractures/dislocations: L clavicle, 1962, fell getting off tractor
Arthritis/unstable joints: "think I've got some in my knees."
Back problems: occ. lower back pain
Vision impaired: requires glasses for reading
Hearing impaired: slightly, compensates by turning "good ear" toward speaker

Reports (Objective)

Temperature: 99.4 oral
Skin integrity: impaired L foot   **Scars:** R Ing, surgical.
Rashes: –0–   **Bruises:** –0–   **Lacerations:** –0–   **Blisters:** –0–
Ulcerations: Medial aspect L foot, 2.5 cm diameter, approx 3 mm deep, draining sm. amt cream color/pink tinged matter, no odor noted.

Strength (general): equal all extremities.   **Muscle tone:** firm
ROM: good   **Gait:** favors L foot   **Paresthesia/Paralysis:** –0–

SEXUALITY: Male

Reports (Subjective)

Penile discharge: –0–   **Prostate disorder:** –0–   **Vasectomy:** –0–
Last proctoscopic exam: 2 yrs ago.   **prostate exam:** 1 yr ago
Practice self-exam: Breast/testicles: No
Problems/complaints: "I don't have any problems, but you'd have to ask my wife if there are any complaints."

Exhibits (Objective)

Exam: Breast: no masses   **Testicles:** deferred   **Prostate:** deferred

SOCIAL INTERACTIONS

Reports (Subjective)

Martial status: married 40 yrs.   **Living with:** wife
Report of problems: None
Extended family: 1 daughter lives in town (30 miles away), 1 daughter married/grandson, living out of state
Other: several couples, he & wife play cards/socialize with 2–3 times/month
Role: works farm alone. Husband/father/grandfather
Report of problems related to illness/condition: none until now.
Coping behaviors: "my wife and I have always talked things out. You know the 11th commandment is Thou shalt not go to bed angry."

Exhibits (Objective)

Speech: clear, intelligible.
Verbal/Non-verbal communication with family /s.o. (s): speaks quietly with wife, looking her in the eye; relaxed posture.
Family interaction patterns: Wife sitting at bedside, relaxed, both reading paper, making occasional comments to each other.

TEACHING/LEARNING

Reports (Subjective)

Dominant language: English   **Literate:** Yes
Education level: 2 years college
Health beliefs/practices: "I take care of the minor problems and only see the doctor when something's broken."
Familial risk factors/relationship:
  Diabetes: Uncle   **Tuberculosis:** brother died age 27
  Heart Disease: f. died, age 78, heart attack
  Strokes: Mo died, age 81   **High B/P:** Mother
Prescribed medications:
Drug: Orinase;   **Dose:** 250   mg   **Schedule:** 8   AM/6   PM, Last   dose   6   PM   today
  Purpose: Diabetes
Home glucose monitoring: "stopped several months ago when I ran out of TesTape. It was always negative anyway."
Does patient take medications regularly? Yes
Non-prescription (OTC) drugs: Occ. ASA
Use of alcohol (amount/frequency): socially, occ. beer

Admitting Diagnosis (physician): Hyperglycemia and L foot ulcer.

Reason for hospitalization (patient): Sore on foot & my sugar is up.

History of current complaint: "3 weeks ago I got a blister on my foot from breaking in my new boots. It got sore so I lanced it but it isn't getting any better."

Patient's expectations of this hospitalization: "Clear up this infection and control my diabetes."

Other relevant illness &/or previous hospitalizations/surgeries: 1965 R Ing. hernia repair

Evidence of failure to improve: lesion L foot, 3 wks.

Last physical exam: complete 1 yr ago, office follow up 3 mos ago.

DISCHARGE CONSIDERATIONS (as of 6/28)

Anticipated discharge: 7/1/87 (3 days)

Resources: Self; wife   **Financial:** "if this doesn't take too long to heal, we got some savings to cover things."

Anticipated lifestyle changes: none

Assistance needed: may require farm help for several days.

Learn new medication regimen and wound care

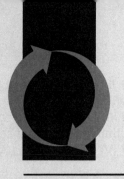

NANDA Nursing Diagnoses with Definitions, Related/Risk Factors, and Defining Characteristics

Activity Intolerance [specify level]

DEFINITION: A state in which an individual has insufficient physiological or psychologic energy to endure or complete required or desired daily activities.

PROBLEM

RELATED FACTORS: ○ Generalized weakness ○ Sedentary lifestyle ○ Bed rest or immobility ○ Imbalance between oxygen supply and demand ○ [Cognitive deficits/emotional status; underlying disease process/depression]

ETIOLOGY

DEFINING CHARACTERISTICS:

SIGNS
AND
SYMPTOMS

    SUBJECTIVE: ■ Verbal report of fatigue or weakness ○ Exertional discomfort or dyspnea ○ [Pain] ○ [Verbalizes no desire and/or lack of interest in activity]

    OBJECTIVE: ○ Abnormal heart rate or blood pressure response ○ Electrocardiographic changes reflecting arrhythmias or ischemia ○ [Pallor] ○ [Cyanosis]

    Suggested levels for determining degree of impairment (Gordon, 1987):

    Level I: walk, regular pace, on level indefinitely; one flight or more but more short of breath than normally

---

■ = critical factors/major signs and symptoms
NOTE: Information appearing in [] has been added by the authors to clarify and facilitate the use of nursing diagnoses.

Level II: walk one city block 500 feet on level; climb one flight slowly without stopping

Level III: walk no more than 50 feet on level without stopping; unable to climb one flight of stairs without stopping

Level IV: dyspnea and fatigue at rest

Activity Intolerance, high risk for*

PROBLEM

DEFINITION: A state in which an individual is at risk of experiencing insufficient physiological or psychologic energy to endure or complete required or desired daily activities.

ETIOLOGY

RISK FACTORS: ○ History of previous intolerance ○ Presence of circulatory/respiratory problems ○ Deconditioned status ○ Presence of circulatory/respiratory problems ○ Inexperience with the activity ○ [Early diagnosis of progressive disease state such as cancer, multiple sclerosis; extensive surgical procedures] ○ [Verbalized reluctance/inability to perform expected activity]

Adjustment, impaired

PROBLEM

DEFINITION: The state in which the individual is unable to modify his/her lifestyle or behavior in a manner consistent with a change in health status.

ETIOLOGY

RELATED FACTORS: ○ Disability requiring change in lifestyle ○ Inadequate support systems ○ Impaired cognition, sensory overload ○ Assault to self-esteem, altered locus of control ○ Incomplete grieving [severe emotional loss] ○ [Physical and/or learning disability] ○ [Life threatening condition or disease]

SIGNS
AND
SYMPTOMS

DEFINING CHARACTERISTICS:

SUBJECTIVE: ■ Verbalization of nonacceptance of health status change

OBJECTIVE: ■ Nonexistent or unsuccessful ability to be involved in problem-solving or goal setting ○ Lack of movement toward independence ○ Extended period of shock, disbelief, or anger regarding health status change ○ Lack of future-oriented thinking ○ [Lack of ability to limit expectations of self]

Airway Clearance, ineffective

PROBLEM

DEFINITION: A state in which an individual is unable to clear secretions or obstructions from the respiratory tract to maintain airway patency.

■ = critical factors/major signs and symptoms

NOTE: Information appearing in [] has been added by the authors to clarify and facilitate the use of nursing diagnoses.

***[NOTE:** A high risk diagnosis is *not* evidenced by signs and symptoms, since the problem has not yet occurred, and nursing interventions are directed at prevention. Therefore, risk factors which are present are noted instead.]

RELATED FACTORS: ○ Tracheobronchial infection, obstruction, secretion ○ Decreased energy/fatigue ○ Perceptual/cognitive impairment ○ Trauma ○ [Inhalation injury]

ETIOLOGY

DEFINING CHARACTERISTICS:

SIGNS
AND
SYMPTOMS

SUBJECTIVE: ○ [Statement of difficulty breathing]

OBJECTIVE: ○ Abnormal breath sounds; rales (crackles), rhonchi (wheezes) ○ Changes in rate or depth of respiration ○ Tachypnea ○ Cough, effective or ineffective, with or without sputum ○ Cyanosis ○ Dyspnea ○ [Apnea] ○ [Fear; anxiety; restlessness] ○ [Use of accessory muscles for breathing] ○ [Choking or noisy respirations]

Anxiety [mild, moderate, severe, panic]

DEFINITION: A vague uneasy feeling whose source is often nonspecific or unknown to the individual.

PROBLEM

RELATED FACTORS: ○ Unconscious conflict about essential values, [beliefs], and goals of life ○ Situational and [or] maturational crises ○ Interpersonal transmission/contagion ○ Threat to self-concept [perceived or actual]; [unconscious conflict] ○ Threat of death [perceived or actual] ○ Threat to or change in health status [terminal illness], role functioning, environment [safety], interaction patterns, socioeconomic status ○ Unmet needs ○ [Positive or negative self-talk] ○ [Physiologic factors, such as hyperthyroidism, pheochromocytoma, use of steroids]

ETIOLOGY

DEFINING CHARACTERISTICS:

SIGNS
AND
SYMPTOMS

SUBJECTIVE: ○ Increased tension ○ Regretful ○ Scared; shakiness ○ Overexcited; rattled; distressed ○ Apprehension; uncertainty; fearful ○ Feelings of inadequacy ○ Fear of unspecific consequences ○ Expressed concern regarding changes in life events ○ Worried; anxious; jittery ○ Painful and persistent increased helplessness ○ [Somatic complaints] ○ [Sleeplessness] ○ [Sense of impending doom] ○ [Hopelessness]

OBJECTIVE: ■ Sympathetic stimulation: cardiovascular excitation, superficial vasoconstriction, pupil dilation ○ Increased wariness; glancing about; poor eye contact ○ Extraneous movements (foot shuffling; hand/arm movements) ○ Increased perspiration ○ Trembling/hand tremors; restlessness ○ Insomnia ○ Facial tension; voice quivering ○ Focus on self ○ [Urinary frequency] ○ [Repetitive questioning] ○ [Pacing/purposeless activity] ○ [Impaired functioning/immobility]

■ = critical factors/major signs and symptoms

NOTE: Information appearing in [] has been added by the authors to clarify and facilitate the use of nursing diagnoses.

Aspiration, high risk for

PROBLEM

DEFINITION: The state in which an individual is at risk for entry of gastric secretions, oropharyngeal secretions, or [exogenous food] solids or fluids into tracheobronchial passages [due to dysfunction or absence of normal protective mechanisms].

ETIOLOGY

RISK FACTORS* ○ Reduced level of consciousness ○ Depressed cough and gag reflexes ○ Impaired swallowing [owing to inability of the epiglottis and true vocal cords to move to close off trachea] ○ Facial/oral/neck surgery or trauma; wired jaws ○ Situation hindering elevation of upper body ○ Delayed gastric emptying; decreased gastrointestinal motility; increased intragastric pressure; increased gastric residual ○ Presence of tracheostomy or endotracheal tube; [over- or inadequate inflation of tracheostomy/endotracheal tube cuff] ○ Gastrointestinal tubes; bolus tube feedings/medication administration

Body Image Disturbance

PROBLEM

DEFINITION: Disruption in the way one perceives one's body image.

ETIOLOGY

RELATED FACTORS: ○ Biophysical [physical trauma/mutilation, pregnancy, physical change caused by biochemical agents (drugs), dependence on machine] ○ Psychosocial ○ Cultural or spiritual ○ (Cognitive/perceptual) ○ (Significance of body part or functioning with regard to age, sex, developmental level, or basic human needs) ○ [Maturational changes]

SIGNS
AND
SYMPTOMS

DEFINING CHARACTERISTICS: ○ *A* or *B* must be present to justify the diagnosis of Body Image disturbance ■ *A* = verbal response to actual or perceived change in structure and/or function ■ *B* = nonverbal response to actual or perceived change in structure and/or function

The following clinical manifestations may be used to validate the presence of *A* or *B*:

SUBJECTIVE: ○ Verbalization of:

Change in lifestyle;
Fear of rejection or of reaction by others;
Focus on past strength, function, or appearance;
Negative feelings about body;
Feelings of helplessness, hopelessness, or powerlessness;
Preoccupation with change or loss; and/or
[Feelings or depersonalization/grandiosity]

○ Refusal to verify actual change ○ Emphasis on remaining strengths, heightened achievement ○ Personalization of part or loss by name ○ Depersonalization of part or loss by impersonal pronouns ○ Extension of body boundary to incorporate environment objects

---

■ = critical factors/major signs and symptoms
NOTE: Information appearing in [] has been added by the authors to clarify and facilitate the use of nursing diagnoses.
*[NOTE: A high risk diagnosis is *not* evidenced by signs and symptoms, since the problem has not yet occurred, and nursing interventions are directed at prevention. Therefore, risk factors which are present are noted instead.]

OBJECTIVE: ○ Missing body part ○ Actual change in structure and/or function ○ Not looking at/not touching body part ○ Trauma to nonfunctioning part ○ Change in ability to estimate spatial relationship of body to environment ○ Hiding or overexposing body part (intentional or unintentional) ○ Change in social involvement ○ [Inability to differentiate internal/external stimuli/loss of ego boundaries]

Body Temperature, altered, high risk for*

DEFINITION: The state in which the individual is at risk for failure to maintain body temperature within normal range.

PROBLEM

RISK FACTORS: ○ Extremes of age, weight ○ Exposure to cold/cool or warm/hot environments ○ Dehydration ○ Inactivity or vigorous activity ○ Medications causing vasoconstriction/vasodilation, altered metabolic rate, sedation, [use or overdose of certain drugs or exposure to anesthesia] ○ Inappropriate clothing for environmental temperature ○ Illness or trauma affecting temperature regulation ○ [Infections, systemic or localized] ○ [Neoplasms, tumors, collagen/vascular disease]

ETIOLOGY

Bowel Incontinence

DEFINITION: A state in which an individual experiences a change in normal bowel habits characterized by involuntary passage of stool.

PROBLEM

RELATED FACTORS: ○ To be developed by NANDA ○ (Neuromuscular/musculoskeletal involvement) ○ (Perceptual or cognitive impairment) ○ (Depression) ○ (Severe anxiety) ○ [Diarrhea and/or fecal impaction]
   Note: These factors were identified when this diagnosis was originally accepted and have been retained here to assist the user until NANDA completes its work.

ETIOLOGY

DEFINING CHARACTERISTICS:
   OBJECTIVE: ○ Involuntary passage of stool

SIGNS
AND
SYMPTOMS

Breastfeeding, effective

DEFINITION: The state in which a mother-infant dyad/family exhibits adequate proficiency and satisfaction with breastfeeding process.

PROBLEM

RELATED FACTORS: ○ Basic breastfeeding knowledge ○ Normal breast structure ○ Normal infant oral structure ○ Infant gestational age greater than 34 weeks ○ Support sources [available] ○ Maternal confidence

ETIOLOGY

■ = critical factors/major signs and symptoms
NOTE: Information appearing in [] has been added by the authors to clarify and facilitate the use of nursing diagnoses.
*[**NOTE:** A high risk diagnosis is *not* evidenced by signs and symptoms, since the problem has not yet occurred, and nursing interventions are directed at prevention. Therefore, risk factors which are present are noted instead.]

SIGNS
AND
SYMPTOMS

DEFINING CHARACTERISTICS:

SUBJECTIVE: ○ Maternal verbalization of satisfaction with the breastfeeding process

OBJECTIVE: ▪ Mother able to position infant at breast to promote a successful latch-on response ▪ Infant is content after feedings ▪ Regular and sustained sucking at the breast (8 to 10 times/24 hours) ▪ Adequate infant weight gain; [appropriate infant weight patterns for age] ○ Signs and/or symptoms of oxytocin release (let down or milk ejection reflex) ○ [Infant] Soft stools; over 6 wet diapers per day of unconcentrated urine; eagerness of infant to nurse

Breastfeeding, ineffective

PROBLEM

DEFINITION: The state in which a mother, infant, or child experiences dissatisfaction or difficulty with the breastfeeding process.

ETIOLOGY

RELATED FACTORS: ○ Prematurity; infant anomaly; poor infant sucking reflex ○ Infant receiving [numerous or repeated] supplemental feedings with artificial nipple ○ Maternal anxiety or ambivalence ○ Knowledge deficit ○ Previous history of breastfeeding failure ○ Interruption in breastfeeding ○ Nonsupportive partner/family ○ Maternal breast anomaly; previous breast surgery; painful nipples/breast engorgement

SIGNS
AND
SYMPTOMS

DEFINING CHARACTERISTICS:

SUBJECTIVE: ▪ Unsatisfactory breastfeeding process ▪ Persistence of sore nipples beyond the first week of breastfeeding ○ Insufficient emptying of each breast per feeding ○ Actual or perceived inadequate milk supply

OBJECTIVE: [▪] Observable signs of inadequate infant intake [inappropriate weight loss/or inadequate gain] ○ Nonsustained or insufficient opportunity for suckling at the breast; infant inability [failure] to attach on to maternal breast correctly ○ Infant arching and crying at the breasts; resisting latching on ○ Infant exhibiting fussiness and crying within the first hour after breastfeeding; unresponsive to other comfort measures ○ No observable signs of oxytocin release

Breathing Pattern, ineffective

PROBLEM

DEFINITION: The state in which an individual's inhalation and/or exhalation pattern does not enable adequate pulmonary inflation or emptying.

ETIOLOGY

RELATED FACTORS: ○ Neuromuscular/musculoskeletal impairment ○ Anxiety ○ Pain ○ Perception/cognitive impairment ○ Decreased energy/fatigue ○ [Alteration of patient's normal 02/CO2 ratio, e.g., 02 therapy in COPD]

SIGNS
AND
SYMPTOMS

DEFINING CHARACTERISTICS:

SUBJECTIVE: ○ Shortness of breath

▪ = critical factors/major signs and symptoms
NOTE: Information appearing in [] has been added by the authors to clarify and facilitate the use of nursing diagnoses.

OBJECTIVE: ○ Dyspnea; tachypnea ○ Fremitus ○ Cough ○ Respiratory depth changes; altered chest excursion ○ Nasal flaring; use of accessory muscles ○ Pursed-lip breathing; prolonged expiratory phase ○ Assumption of three-point position ○ Cyanosis; abnormal arterial blood gas ○ Increased anteroposterior diameter ○ [Reduced vital capacity] ○ [Tachycardia]

Cardiac Output, decreased

DEFINITION: A state in which the blood pumped by an individual's heart is sufficiently reduced that it is inadequate to meet the needs of the body's tissues. [*Note:* In a hypermetabolic state, although cardiac output may be within normal range, it may still be inadequate to meet the needs of the body's tissues. Cardiac output and tissue perfusion are interrelated although there are differences. When cardiac output is decreased, tissue perfusion problems will develop; however, tissue perfusion problems can exist without decreased cardiac output.] — PROBLEM

RELATED FACTORS: ○ To be developed by NANDA ○ (Mechanical: alteration in preload [e.g., decreased venous return, altered myocardial contractility]; afterload [e.g., alteration in systemic vascular resistance]; inotropic changes in heart) ○ (Electrical: alterations in rate; rhythm; conduction) ○ (Structural [e.g., ventricular-septal rupture, ventricular aneurysm, papillary muscle rupture, valvular disease]) — ETIOLOGY

Note: These factors were identified when the diagnosis was originally accepted and have been retained here to assist the user until NANDA completes its work.

DEFINING CHARACTERISTICS: — SIGNS AND SYMPTOMS

SUBJECTIVE: ○ Fatigue ○ Dyspnea

OBJECTIVE: ○ Variations in blood pressure [and hemodynamic] readings ○ Color changes, skin and mucous membranes [cyanosis] ○ Cold, clammy skin ○ Orthopnea ○ Arrhythmias; [ECG changes] ○ Jugular vein distention ○ Oliguria; anuria ○ Decreased peripheral pulses ○ Rales ○ Restlessness

OTHER POSSIBLE CHARACTERISTICS:

SUBJECTIVE ○ Syncope ○ Vertigo ○ Weakness ○ [Angina]

OBJECTIVE: ○ Edema ○ Change in mental status ○ Shortness of breath ○ Frothy sputum ○ Gallop rhythm; abnormal heart sounds ○ Cough ○ [Liver engorgement/ascites]

Communication, impaired verbal

DEFINITION: The state in which an individual experiences a decreased or absent ability to use or understand language in human interaction. — PROBLEM

■ = critical factors/major signs and symptoms
NOTE: Information appearing in [] has been added by the authors to clarify and facilitate the use of nursing diagnoses.

ETIOLOGY

RELATED FACTORS: ○ Decrease in circulation to brain; brain tumor ○ Anatomic deficit, cleft palate ○ Development or age-related ○ Physical barrier (tracheostomy, intubation) ○ Psychologic barriers (psychosis, lack of stimuli, [depression, panic, anger]) ○ Cultural difference ○ [Drug intake; chemical imbalance]

SIGNS
AND
SYMPTOMS

DEFINING CHARACTERISTICS:

SUBJECTIVE: ○ [Reports of difficulty expressing self]

OBJECTIVE: ■ Unable to speak dominant language ■ Speaks or verbalizes with difficulty ■ Does not or cannot speak ○ Disorientation ○ Stuttering; slurring ○ Dyspnea ○ Difficulty forming words or sentences ○ Difficulty expressing thought verbally ○ Inappropriate verbalization, [incessant, loose association of ideas, flight of ideas] ○ [Inability to modulate speech] ○ [Message inappropriate to content] ○ [Use of nonverbal cues, e.g., facial expression, gestures, pleading eyes, turning away] ○ [Frustration, anger, hostility]

Constipation

PROBLEM

DEFINITION: A state in which an individual experiences a change in normal bowel habits characterized by a decrease in frequency and/or passage of hard, dry stools.

ETIOLOGY

RELATED FACTORS: ○ To be developed by NANDA ○ (Neuromuscular/Musculoskeletal impairment, weak abdominal musculature) ○ (Gastrointestinal obstructive lesions) ○ (Pain on defecation) ○ (Diagnostic procedures) ○ (Pregnancy)

Note: These factors were identified when this diagnosis was originally accepted and have been retained here to assist the user until NANDA completes its work.

SIGNS
AND
SYMPTOMS

DEFINING CHARACTERISTICS:

SUBJECTIVE: ○ Frequency less than usual pattern ○ Reported feeling of abdominal or rectal fullness or pressure ○ [Less than usual amount of stool] ○ [Nausea]

OBJECTIVE: ○ Hard-formed stools ○ Straining at stool ○ Palpable mass ○ Decreased activity level ○ [Decreased bowel sounds] ○ [Abdominal distention] ○ Other possible characteristics:

Abdominal/back pain;
Headache;
Interference with daily living;
Appetite impairment; and/or
Use of laxatives

■ = critical factors/major signs and symptoms
NOTE: Information appearing in [] has been added by the authors to clarify and facilitate the use of nursing diagnoses.

Constipation, colonic

DEFINITION: The state in which an individual's pattern of elimination is characterized by hard, dry stool which results from a delay in passage of food residue.

PROBLEM

RELATED FACTORS: ○ Less than adequate fluid/dietary intake; less than adequate fiber ○ Less than adequate physical activity; immobility ○ Lack of privacy; emotional disturbances; stress; change in daily routine ○ Chronic use of medication and enemas ○ Metabolic problems, for example, hypothyroidism, hypocalcemia, hypokalemia

ETIOLOGY

DEFINING CHARACTERISTICS ■ Hard, dry stool ■ Decreased frequency ■ Straining at stool ■ Painful defecation ■ Abdominal distention ■ Palpable mass ○ Abdominal pain ○ Rectal pressure ○ Appetite impairment ○ Headache

SIGNS
AND
SYMPTOMS

Constipation, perceived

DEFINITION: The state in which an individual makes a self-diagnosis of constipation and ensures a daily bowel movement through use of laxatives, enemas, and suppositories.

PROBLEM

RELATED FACTORS: ○ Cultural/family health benefits ○ Faulty appraisal ○ Impaired thought processes

ETIOLOGY

DEFINING CHARACTERISTICS ■ Expectation of a daily bowel movement with the resulting overuse of laxatives, enemas, and suppositories ■ Expected passage of stool at same time every day

SIGNS
AND
SYMPTOMS

Coping, defensive

DEFINITION: The state in which an individual repeatedly projects falsely positive self-evaluation based on a self-protective pattern which defends against underlying perceived threats to positive self-regard.

PROBLEM

RELATED FACTORS: ○ Refer to ND Coping, ineffective, individual.

ETIOLOGY

DEFINING CHARACTERISTICS:

SIGNS
AND
SYMPTOMS

SUBJECTIVE: ■ Denial of obvious problems/weaknesses ■ Projection of blame/responsibility ■ Hypersensitive to slight/criticism ■ Grandiosity ○ Rationalizes failures

OBJECTIVE: ○ Superior attitude toward others ○ Difficulty establishing/maintaining relationships ○ Hostile laughter or ridicule of others ○ Difficulty in reality testing perceptions ○ Lack of follow-through or participation in treatment or therapy

---

■ = critical factors/major signs and symptoms
NOTE: Information appearing in [] has been added by the authors to clarify and facilitate the use of nursing diagnoses.

Coping, ineffective, individual

PROBLEM

DEFINITION: Impairment of adaptive behaviors and problem-solving abilities of a person in meeting life's demands and roles.

ETIOLOGY

RELATED FACTORS: ○ Situational/maturational crises ○ Personal vulnerability ○ Inadequate support systems ○ Poor nutrition ○ Work overload; no vacations; [too many deadlines] ○ Unrealistic perceptions ○ [Multiple stressors, repeated over period of time] ○ [Multiple life changes; conflict] ○ [Inadequate relaxation, little or no exercise] ○ [Unmet expectations] ○ [Inadequate coping method] ○ [Impairment of nervous system] ○ [Memory loss] ○ [Severe pain, overwhelming threat to self]

SIGNS
AND
SYMPTOMS

DEFINING CHARACTERISTICS:

SUBJECTIVE ■ Verbalization of inability to cope or inability to ask for help ○ Reports of chronic worry/anxiety/depression, poor self-esteem ○ [Complaints of muscular/emotional tension, lack of appetite, chronic fatigue, insomnia, general irritability]

OBJECTIVE: ■ Inability to problem-solve ○ Inability to meet role expectations/basic needs ○ Alteration in societal participation ○ Inappropriate use of defense mechanisms ○ Change in usual communication patterns ○ Verbal manipulation ○ High illness rate [including high blood pressure, ulcers, irritable bowel, frequent headaches/neckaches] ○ High rate of accidents ○ Destructive behavior toward self or others [including overeating, excessive smoking/drinking, overuse of prescribed tranquilizers, alcohol] ○ [Lack of assertive behaviors]

Decisional Conflict [specify]

PROBLEM

DEFINITION: The state of uncertainty about course of action to be taken when choice among competing actions involves risk, loss, or challenge to personal life values.

ETIOLOGY

RELATED FACTORS: ○ Unclear personal values/beliefs; perceived threat to value system ○ Lack of experience or interference with decision-making ○ Lack of relevant information; multiple or divergent sources of information ○ Support system deficit

SIGNS
AND
SYMPTOMS

DEFINING CHARACTERISTICS:

SUBJECTIVE ■ Verbalized uncertainty about choices or of undesired consequences of alternative actions being considered ○ Verbalized feelings of distress or questioning personal values and beliefs while attempting a decision

OBJECTIVE: ■ Vacillation between alternative choices; delayed decision-making ○ Self-focusing ○ Physical signs of distress or tension (increased heart rate; increased muscle tension; restlessness etc.)

■ = critical factors/major signs and symptoms
NOTE: Information appearing in [] has been added by the authors to clarify and facilitate the use of nursing diagnoses.

Denial, ineffective

DEFINITION: The state of a conscious or unconscious attempt to disavow the knowledge or meaning of an event to reduce anxiety/fear to the detriment of health.

PROBLEM

RELATED FACTORS: ○ To be developed by NANDA ○ [Personal vulnerability; unmet self-needs] ○ [Presence of overwhelming anxiety-producing feelings/situation; reality factors that are consciously intolerable]

ETIOLOGY

DEFINING CHARACTERISTICS:

SIGNS
AND
SYMPTOMS

SUBJECTIVE: ○ Minimizes symptoms; displaces source of symptoms to other organs ○ Unable to admit impact of disease on life pattern ○ Displaces fear of impact of the condition ○ Does not admit fear of death or invalidism

OBJECTIVE: ■ Delays seeking or refuses healthcare attention to the detriment of health ■ Does not perceive personal relevance of symptoms or danger ○ Makes dismissive gestures or comments when speaking of distressing events ○ Displays inappropriate affect ○ Uses home remedies (self-treatment) to relieve symptoms

Diarrhea

DEFINITION: A state in which an individual experiences a change in normal bowel habits characterized by the frequent passage of loose, fluid, unformed stools.

PROBLEM

RELATED FACTORS: ○ To be developed by NANDA ○ (Stress and anxiety) ○ (Medications, radiation, toxins, contaminants) ○ (Dietary intake) ○ (Inflammation, irritation, or malabsorption of bowel)

ETIOLOGY

Note: These factors were identified when this diagnosis was originally accepted and have been retained here to assist the user until NANDA completes its work.

DEFINING CHARACTERISTICS:

SIGNS
AND
SYMPTOMS

SUBJECTIVE: ○ Abdominal pain ○ Urgency; cramping

OBJECTIVE: ○ Increased frequency ○ Increased frequency of bowel sounds ○ Loose, liquid stools

OTHER POSSIBLE CHARACTERISTICS: ○ Change in color

Disuse Syndrome, high risk for*

DEFINITION: A state in which an individual is at risk for deterioration of body systems as the result of prescribed or unavoidable musculoskeletal inactivity.

PROBLEM

■ = critical factors/major signs and symptoms

NOTE: Information appearing in [] has been added by the authors to clarify and facilitate the use of nursing diagnoses.

*[**NOTE:** A high risk diagnosis is *not* evidenced by signs and symptoms, since the problem has not yet occurred, and nursing interventions are directed at prevention. Therefore, risk factors which are present are noted instead.]

(*Note:* NANDA identifies complications from immobility including pressure ulcer, constipation, stasis of pulmonary secretions, thrombosis, urinary tract infection/retention, decreased strength/endurance, orthostatic hypotension, decreased range of joint motion, disorientation, body image disturbance, and powerlessness.)

ETIOLOGY

RISK FACTORS:

SUBJECTIVE: ○ Severe pain, [chronic pain]

OBJECTIVE: ○ Paralysis ○ Mechanical or prescribed immobilization ○ Altered level of consciousness

---

Diversional Activity Deficit

PROBLEM

DEFINITION: The state in which an individual experiences a decreased stimulation from or interest or engagement in recreational or leisure activities. [*Note:* Internal/external factors may or may not be beyond the individual's control.]

ETIOLOGY

RELATED FACTORS: ○ Environmental lack of diversional activity, for example, long-term hospitalization; frequent, lengthy treatments ○ [Physical limitations, bedridden] ○ [Situation, development problem] ○ [Psychologic condition, e.g., depression]

SIGNS AND SYMPTOMS

DEFINING CHARACTERISTICS:

SUBJECTIVE: ○ Patient's statement regarding the following:

Boredom; Wish there were something to do, to read, etc.;
Usual hobbies cannot be undertaken in hospital [or are restricted by physical limitations]

OBJECTIVE: ○ [Flat affect; disinterested] ○ [Restless; crying] ○ [Lethargy; withdrawn] ○ [Hostile]

Dysreflexia

PROBLEM

DEFINITION: The state in which an individual with a spinal cord injury at T7 or above experiences a life threatening uninhibited sympathetic response of the nervous system to a noxious stimulus.

ETIOLOGY

RELATED FACTORS: ○ Bladder or bowel distention ○ Skin irritation ○ Lack of patient and caregiver knowledge ○ [Sexual excitation]

SIGNS AND SYMPTOMS

DEFINING CHARACTERISTICS ■ Individual with spinal cord injury (T7 or above) with:

SUBJECTIVE: ■ Headache (a diffuse pain in different portions of the head and not confined to any nerve distribution area) ○ Paresthesia; chilling; blurred vision; chest pain; metallic taste in mouth; nasal congestion ○ Pilomotor reflex (gooseflesh formation such as when skin is cooled)

■ = critical factors/major signs and symptoms
NOTE: Information appearing in [] has been added by the authors to clarify and facilitate the use of nursing diagnoses.

OBJECTIVE: ■ Paroxysmal hypertension (sudden periodic elevated blood pressure where systolic pressure is over 140 mmHg and diastolic is above 90 mmHg) ■ Bradycardia or tachycardia (pulse rate of less than 60 or over 100 beats per minute) ■ Diaphoresis (above the injury); red splotches on skin (above the injury); pallor (below the injury) ○ Horner's syndrome (contraction of the pupil, partial ptosis of the eyelid, enophthalmos and sometimes loss of sweating over the affected side of the face); conjunctival congestion

Family Coping, compromised

DEFINITION: A usually supportive primary person (family member or close friend [significant other]) is providing insufficient, ineffective, or compromised support, comfort, assistance, or encouragement which may be needed by the client to manage or master adaptive tasks related to his or her health challenge.

PROBLEM

RELATED FACTORS: ○ Inadequate or incorrect information or understanding by a primary person ○ Temporary preoccupation by a significant person who is trying to manage emotional conflicts and personal suffering and is unable to perceive or act effectively in regard to client's needs ○ Temporary family disorganization and role changes ○ Other situation or development crises or situations the significant person may by facing ○ Little support provided by client, in turn, for primary person ○ Prolonged disease or disability progressing that exhausts the supportive capacity of significant people

ETIOLOGY

DEFINING CHARACTERISTICS:

SUBJECTIVE: ○ Client expresses or confirms a concern or complaint about significant other's response to his or her health problem ○ Significant person describes preoccupation with personal reaction (e.g., fear, anticipatory grief, guilt, anxiety) to client's illness/disability, or to other situation or development crises ○ Significant person describes or confirms an inadequate understanding or knowledge base which interferes with effective assistive or supportive behaviors.

SIGNS AND SYMPTOMS

OBJECTIVE: ○ Significant person attempts assistive or supportive behaviors with less than satisfactory results ○ Significant person withdraws or enters into limited or temporary personal communication with client at the time of need ○ Significant person displays protective behavior disproportionate (too little or too much) to client's abilities or need for autonomy

Family Coping, disabling

DEFINITION: Behavior of significant person (family member or other primary person) that disables his or her own capacities and the client's capacities to effectively address tasks essential to either person's adaptation to the health challenge.

PROBLEM

■ = critical factors/major signs and symptoms
NOTE: Information appearing in [] has been added by the authors to clarify and facilitate the use of nursing diagnoses.

ETIOLOGY

RELATED FACTORS: ○ Significant person with chronically unexpressed feelings of guilt, anxiety, hostility, despair, etc. ○ Dissonant discrepancy of coping styles for dealing with adaptive tasks by the significant person and client or among significant people ○ Highly ambivalent family relationships ○ Arbitrary handling of a family's resistance to treatment, which tends to solidify defensiveness as it fails to deal adequately with underlying anxiety

SIGNS
AND
SYMPTOMS

DEFINING CHARACTERISTICS:

    SUBJECTIVE: ○ [Expresses despair re family reactions/lack of involvement]

    OBJECTIVE: ○ Intolerance; abandonment; rejection; desertion ○ Psychosomaticism ○ Agitation, depression, aggression, hostility ○ Taking on illness signs of the client ○ Neglectful relationships with other family members ○ Carrying on usual routines disregarding client's needs ○ Neglectful care of the client in regard to basic human needs and/or illness treatment ○ Distortion of reality regarding the client's health problem, including extreme denial about its existence or severity ○ Decisions and actions by family which are detrimental to economic or social well-being ○ Impaired restructuring of a meaningful life for self, impaired individualization, prolonged overconcern for client ○ Client's development of helpless, inactive dependence

---

Family Coping, potential for growth

PROBLEM

DEFINITION: Effective managing of adaptive tasks by family member involved with the client's health challenge, who now is exhibiting desire and readiness for enhanced health and growth in regard to self and in relation to the client.

ETIOLOGY

RELATED FACTORS: ○ Needs sufficiently gratified and adaptive tasks effectively addressed to enable goals of self-actualization to surface

SIGNS
AND
SYMPTOMS

DEFINING CHARACTERISTICS:

    SUBJECTIVE: ○ Family member attempting to describe growth impact of crisis on his/her own values, priorities, goals, or relationships ○ Individual expressing interest in making contact on a one-to-one basis or on a mutual-aid group basis with another person who has experienced a similar situation

    OBJECTIVE: ○ Family member moving in direction of health-promoting and enriching lifestyle which supports and monitors maturational processes, audits and negotiates treatment programs, and generally chooses experiences which optimize wellness

---

Family Processes, altered

PROBLEM

DEFINITION: The state in which a family that normally functions effectively experiences a dysfunction.

■ = critical factors/major signs and symptoms
NOTE: Information appearing in [] has been added by the authors to clarify and facilitate the use of nursing diagnoses.

RELATED FACTORS: ○ Situation transition and/or crises [e.g., economic, change in roles, illness] ○ Development transition and/or crises [e.g., loss or gain of a family member]

ETIOLOGY

DEFINING CHARACTERISTICS:

SIGNS
AND
SYMPTOMS

SUBJECTIVE: ○ Family uninvolved in community activities ○ Unexamined family myths ○ [Family expresses confusion about what to do, verbalizes they are having difficulty coping with situation]

OBJECTIVE: ○ Family system unable to [does not] meet physical/emotional/spiritual needs of its members ○ Family unable to [does not] meet security needs of its members ○ Inability to accept or receive help appropriately ○ Family unable to [does not] adapt to change or to deal with traumatic experience constructively ○ Parents do not demonstrate respect for each other's views on child-rearing practices ○ Inability to express/accept wide range of feelings/feelings of family members ○ Inability of family members to relate to each other for mutual growth and maturation ○ Rigidity in function and roles ○ Family does not demonstrate respect for individuality and autonomy of its members ○ Family failing to accomplish current/past development task ○ Unhealthy family decision-making process ○ Failure to send and receive clear messages ○ Inappropriate level and direction of energy ○ Inappropriate boundary maintenance ○ Inappropriate/poorly communicated family rules, rituals, symbols

Fatigue

DEFINITION: An overwhelming sustained sense of exhaustion and decreased capacity for physical and mental work.

PROBLEM

RELATED FACTORS: ○ Decreased/increased metabolic energy production; altered body chemistry (e.g., medications; drug withdrawal/chemotherapy); increased energy requirements to perform activity of daily living ○ Overwhelming psychologic or emotional demands; excessive social and/or role demands; states of discomfort

ETIOLOGY

DEFINING CHARACTERISTICS:

SIGNS
AND
SYMPTOMS

SUBJECTIVE: ■ Verbalization of an unremitting and overwhelming lack of energy; inability to maintain usual routines ○ Perceived need for additional energy to accomplish routine tasks ○ Impaired ability to concentrate ○ Decreased libido

OBJECTIVE: ○ Increase in physical complaints ○ Emotionally labile or irritable ○ Lethargic or listless; disinterest in surroundings/introspection ○ Decreased performance; accident prone

■ = critical factors/major signs and symptoms
NOTE: Information appearing in [] has been added by the authors to clarify and facilitate the use of nursing diagnoses.

Fear

PROBLEM

DEFINITION: Feeling of dread related to an identifiable source which the person validates.

ETIOLOGY

RELATED FACTORS: ○ To be developed by NANDA ○ (Natural or innate origins: environmental stimuli (e.g., sudden noise), loss of physical support, heights, pain) ○ (Learned response: conditioning, modeling from or identification with others) ○ (Separation from support system in a potentially threatening situation such as hospitalization, treatments, etc.) ○ (Knowledge deficit or unfamiliarity) ○ (Phobic stimulus or phobia) ○ (Language barrier) [/inability to communicate] ○ (Sensory impairment) ○ [Threat of death, perceived or actual]

Note: These factors were identified when this diagnosis was originally accepted and have been retained here to assist the user until NANDA completes its work.

SIGNS
AND
SYMPTOMS

DEFINING CHARACTERISTICS:

SUBJECTIVE: [■] Ability to identify object of fear ○ Panic; scared; jittery ○ [Increased tension; apprehension; frightened; terrified] ○ [Impulsiveness] ○ [Decreased self-assurance] ○ [Associated physical symptoms; nausea, "heart beating fast," etc.]

OBJECTIVE: ○ [Attack/fight behavior—aggressive; flight behavior—withdrawal] ○ [Wide-eyed; increased alertness; concentration on source] ○ [Sympathetic stimulation: cardiovascular excitation, superficial vasoconstriction, pupil dilation, vomiting, diarrhea, diaphoresis, etc.]

Fluid Volume Deficit [active loss]†

PROBLEM

DEFINITION: The state in which an individual experiences vascular, cellular, or intracellular dehydration [in excess of needs or replacement capabilities due to active loss].

ETIOLOGY

RELATED FACTORS: ○ Active loss [e.g., burns, abdominal cancer, hemorrhage, diarrhea, fistulas. Use of hyperosmotic radiopaque contrast agents.]

SIGNS
AND
SYMPTOMS

DEFINING CHARACTERISTICS:

OBJECTIVE: ○ Decreased urine output ○ Output greater than intake ○ Decreased venous filling ○ Increased serum sodium ○ Concentrated urine ○ Sudden weight loss ○ Hemoconcentration

OTHER DEFINING CHARACTERISTICS ○ Hypotension [postural] ○ Thirst ○ Increased pulse rate ○ Decreased skin turgor ○ Decreased pulse volume and pressure ○ Change in mental state ○ Increased body temperature ○ Dry skin/mucous membranes ○ Weakness

---

■ = critical factors/major signs and symptoms
NOTE: Information appearing in [] has been added by the authors to clarify and facilitate the use of nursing diagnoses.
† Note: NANDA has combined the originally individual diagnoses of Fluid volume, deficit, Regulatory Failure and Active Loss. As the etiology and some interventions for these two diagnoses differ, we have chosen to leave them separate.

Fluid Volume Deficit, high risk for*

DEFINITION: The state in which an individual is at risk of experiencing vascular, cellular, or intracellular dehydration [due to active or regulatory losses of body water in excess of needs or replacement capability].

PROBLEM

RISK FACTORS: ○ Extremes of age and weight ○ Loss of fluid through abnormal routes, for example, indwelling tubes ○ Knowledge deficiency related to fluid volume ○ Factors influencing fluid needs, for example, hypermetabolic states ○ Medications, for example, diuretics ○ Excessive losses through normal routes, for example, diarrhea ○ Deviations affecting access to, intake of, or absorption of fluids, for example, physical immobility

ETIOLOGY

Fluid Volume Deficit [regulatory failure]†

DEFINITION: The state in which an individual experiences vascular, cellular, or intracellular dehydration [in excess of needs or replacement capabilities due to failure of regulatory mechanisms].

PROBLEM

RELATED FACTORS: ○ Failure of regulator mechanisms [e.g., adrenal disease, recovery phase of acute renal failure, uncontrolled diabetes mellitus/insipidus]

ETIOLOGY

DEFINING CHARACTERISTICS:

SIGNS
AND
SYMPTOMS

SUBJECTIVE: ○ [Complaints of fatigue, nervousness]

OBJECTIVE: ○ Increased urine output ○ Dilute urine ○ Sudden weight loss ○ Decreased venous filling ○ Hemoconcentration ○ Altered serum sodium

OTHER DEFINING CHARACTERISTICS: ○ Hypotension [postural] ○ Thirst ○ Increased pulse rate ○ Decreased skin turgor ○ Decreased pulse volume and pressure ○ Change in mental status ○ Increased body temperature ○ Dry skin/mucous membranes ○ Weakness ○ [Edema; possible weight gain]

Fluid Volume, excess

DEFINITION: The state in which an individual experiences increased fluid retention and edema.

PROBLEM

RELATED FACTORS: ○ Compromised regulatory mechanism [e.g., SIADH or decreased plasma proteins, e.g., malnutrition, draining fistulas, burns, organ failure] ○ Excess fluid intake ○ Excess sodium intake ○ [Drug therapies: e.g., chlorpropamide, tolbutamide, vincristine, triptyline, carbamazepine]

ETIOLOGY

■ = critical factors/major signs and symptoms
NOTE: Information appearing in [] has been added by the authors to clarify and facilitate the use of nursing diagnoses.
***[NOTE:** A high risk diagnosis is not evidenced by signs and symptoms, since the problem has not yet occurred, and nursing interventions are directed at prevention. Therefore, risk factors which are present are noted instead.]
† Note: NANDA has combined the originally individual diagnoses of Fluid volume, deficit, Regulatory Failure and Active Loss. As the etiology and some interventions for these two diagnoses differ, we have chosen to leave them separate.

SIGNS
AND
SYMPTOMS

DEFINING CHARACTERISTICS:

    SUBJECTIVE: ○ Shortness of breath, orthopnea ○ Anxiety

    OBJECTIVE: ○ Edema; effusion; anasarca ○ Weight gain ○ Intake greater than output ○ Third heart sound (S3) ○ Pulmonary congestion (chest x-ray) ○ Abnormal breath sounds, rales (crackles) ○ Change in respiratory pattern ○ Change in mental status; restlessness ○ Blood pressure changes ○ Central venous pressure changes ○ Pulmonary artery pressure changes ○ Jugular venous distention ○ Positive hepatojugular reflex ○ Oliguria; specific gravity changes ○ Azotemia; altered electrolytes ○ Decreased hemoglobin, hematocrit

Gas Exchange, impaired

PROBLEM

DEFINITION: The state in which the individual experiences a decreased passage of oxygen and/or carbon dioxide between the alveoli of the lungs and the vascular system. [This may be an entity of its own but may also be an end result of other pathology with an interrelatedness between airway clearance and/or breathing pattern problems.]

ETIOLOGY

RELATED FACTORS: ○ Ventilation perfusion imbalance ○ [Altered blood flow, e.g., pulmonary embolus, increased vascular resistance] ○ [Alveolar-capillary membrane changes, e.g., adult respiratory distress syndrome; chronic conditions, such as pneumonoconiosis, asbestosis/silicosis] ○ [Altered oxygen supply, e.g., altitude sickness] ○ [Altered oxygen-carrying capacity of blood, e.g., Sickle cell/other anemia, carbon monoxide poisoning]

SIGNS
AND
SYMPTOMS

DEFINING CHARACTERISTICS:

    SUBJECTIVE: ○ [Dyspnea] ○ [Sense of impending doom]

    OBJECTIVE: ○ Confusion ○ Restlessness ○ Inability to move secretions ○ Hypoxia ○ Somnolence ○ Irritability ○ Hypercapnea ○ [Cyanosis] ○ [Tachycardia] ○ [Polycythemia]

Grieving, anticipatory

PROBLEM

DEFINITION: [Response to loss before it actually occurs. *Note:* May be a healthy response requiring interventions of support and information-giving.]

ETIOLOGY

RELATED FACTORS: ○ To be developed by NANDA ○ [Perceived potential loss of: significant other, physiopsychosocial well-being, personal possessions]

SIGNS
AND
SYMPTOMS

DEFINING CHARACTERISTICS:

    SUBJECTIVE: ○ Sorrow; guilt; anger; choked feelings ○ Denial of potential loss ○ Expression of distress at potential loss ○ Alterations in activity level; sleep patterns ○ Changes in eating habits ○ Altered libido

---

■ = critical factors/major signs and symptoms
NOTE: Information appearing in [] has been added by the authors to clarify and facilitate the use of nursing diagnoses.

OBJECTIVE: ○ Potential loss of significant object ○ Altered communication patterns ○ [Altered affect] ○ [Crying]

Grieving, dysfunctional

DEFINITION: [Delayed or exaggerated response to a perceived, actual, or potential loss.]

PROBLEM

RELATED FACTORS: ○ Actual or perceived object loss (*object loss* is used in the broadest sense). Objects may include people, possessions, a job, status, home, ideals, parts and processes of the body [e.g., amputation, paralysis, chronic/fatal illness]. ○ [Thwarted grieving response to a loss] ○ [Lack of resolution of previous grieving response] ○ [Absence of anticipatory grieving]

ETIOLOGY

DEFINING CHARACTERISTICS:

SUBJECTIVE: ○ Verbal expression of distress at loss ○ Expression of unresolved issues ○ Idealization of lost object ○ Denial of loss ○ Anger; sadness ○ Alterations in: eating habits, sleep and dream patterns, activity levels, libido ○ Reliving of past experiences ○ Expression of guilt ○ [Hopelessness]

SIGNS
AND
SYMPTOMS

OBJECTIVE: ○ Crying ○ Difficulty in expressing loss ○ Interference with life functioning ○ Alterations in concentration and/or pursuits of tasks ○ Labile affect ○ Development regression ○ [Isolation]

Growth and Development, altered

DEFINITION: The state in which an individual demonstrates deviations in norms from his/her age group.

PROBLEM

RELATED FACTORS: ○ Inadequate caretaking; [physical/emotional neglect/abuse] ○ Indifference, inconsistent responsiveness, multiple caretakers ○ Separation from significant other(s) ○ Environmental and stimulation deficiencies ○ Effects of physical disability [handicapping condition] ○ Prescribed dependence [insufficient expectations for self-care]

ETIOLOGY

DEFINING CHARACTERISTICS:

SUBJECTIVE: ■ Delay or difficulty in performing skills (motor, social, or expressive) typical of age group ■ Altered physical growth ■ Inability to perform self-care or self-control activities appropriate for age ■ Loss of previously acquired skills; precocious or accelerated skill attainment]

SIGNS
AND
SYMPTOMS

OBJECTIVE: ○ Flat affect ○ Listlessness, decreased responses

Health Maintenance, altered

DEFINITION: Inability to identify, manage, and/or seek out help to maintain health. [This diagnosis contains components of other nursing diagnoses. We

PROBLEM

■ = critical factors/major signs and symptoms
NOTE: Information appearing in [] has been added by the authors to clarify and facilitate the use of nursing diagnoses.

recommend subsuming health maintenance interventions under the "basic" nursing diagnosis when a single causative factor is identified, e.g., Knowledge Deficit; Communication, impaired, verbal; Thought Processes, altered; Individual/Family Coping, ineffective.]

ETIOLOGY

RELATED FACTORS: ○ Lack of or significant alteration in communication skills (written, verbal, and/or gestural) ○ Unachieved development tasks ○ Lack of ability to make deliberate and thoughtful judgments ○ Perceptual or cognitive impairment (complete or partial lack of gross and/or fine motor skills) ○ Ineffective individual coping; dysfunctional grieving ○ Ineffective family coping; disabling spiritual distress ○ Lack of material resource

SIGNS
AND
SYMPTOMS

DEFINING CHARACTERISTICS:

SUBJECTIVE: ○ Expressed interest in improving health behaviors ○ Reported or observed lack of equipment, financial, and/or other resources ○ Reported or observed impairment of personal support system

OBJECTIVE: ○ Demonstrated lack of knowledge regarding basic health practices ○ Reported or observed inability to take the responsibility for meeting basic health practices in any or all functional pattern areas ○ Demonstrated lack of adaptive behaviors to internal/external environmental changes ○ History of lack of health seeking behavior

Health-Seeking Behaviors (specify)

PROBLEM

DEFINITION: A state in which an individual in stable health is actively seeking ways to alter personal health habits and/or the environment in order to move toward higher level of health. (Stable health status is defined as age appropriate illness prevention measures achieved, client reports good or excellent health, and signs and symptoms of disease if present are controlled.)

ETIOLOGY

RELATED FACTORS: ○ [Situation/maturation occurrence precipitating concern about current health status)

SIGNS
AND
SYMPTOMS

DEFINING CHARACTERISTICS:

SUBJECTIVE: ■ Expressed desire to seek a higher level of wellness ■ Expressed desire to modify codependent behaviors ○ Expressed desire for increased control of health practice ○ Expression of concern about current environmental conditions on health status ○ Stated (or observed) unfamiliarity with wellness community resources

OBJECTIVE: ■ Observed desire to seek a higher level of wellness ○ Observed desire for increased control of health practice ○ Demonstrated or observed lack of knowledge in health promotion behaviors

---

■ = critical factors/major signs and symptoms
NOTE: Information appearing in [] has been added by the authors to clarify and facilitate the use of
    nursing diagnoses.

Home Maintenance Management, impaired

DEFINITION: Inability to independently maintain a safe, growth promoting immediate environment.　　　　　　　　　　　　　　　PROBLEM

RELATED FACTORS: ○ Individual/family member disease or injury ○ Insuffi-　ETIOLOGY
cient family organization or planning ○ Insufficient finances ○ Impaired cognitive or emotional functioning ○ Lack of role modeling ○ Unfamiliarity with
neighborhood resources ○ Lack of knowledge ○ Inadequate support systems

DEFINING CHARACTERISTICS:　　　　　　　　　　　　　　SIGNS
　　　SUBJECTIVE: ■ Household members express difficulty in maintaining their　AND
home in a comfortable fashion ■ Household requests assistance with home　SYMPTOMS
maintenance ■ Household members describe outstanding debts or financial
crises

　　　OBJECTIVE: ■ Accumulation of dirt, food, or hygienic wastes ■ Unwashed
or unavailable cooking equipment, clothes, or linen ■ Overtaxed family members, for example, exhausted, anxious ■ Repeated hygienic disorders, infesta-
tions, or infections ○ Disorderly surroundings ○ Inappropriate household
temperature ○ Lack of necessary equipment or aids ○ Presence of vermin or
rodents ○ Offensive odors

Hopelessness

DEFINITION: A subjective state in which an individual sees limited or no　PROBLEM
alternatives or personal choices available and is unable to mobilize energy on
own behalf.

RELATED FACTORS: ○ Prolonged activity restriction creating isolation ○ Fail-　ETIOLOGY
ing or deteriorating physiologic condition ○ Long-term stress; abandonment ○ Lost belief in transcendent values/God

DEFINING CHARACTERISTICS:　　　　　　　　　　　　　　SIGNS
　　　SUBJECTIVE: ■ Verbal cues (despondent content, "I can't," sighing)　AND
　　　OBJECTIVE: ■ Passivity, decreased verbalization ■ Decreased affect ○　SYMPTOMS
Lack of initiative ○ Decreased response to stimuli ○ Turning away from
speaker ○ Closing eyes ○ Shrugging in response to speaker ○ Decreased appetite, increased/decreased sleep ○ Lack of involvement in care/passively
allowing care [■] Withdrawal from environs ○ [Lack of involvement/interest
in significant other(s) (children, spouse)]

Hyperthermia

DEFINITION: A state in which an individual's body temperature is elevated　PROBLEM
above his/her normal range.

■ = critical factors/major signs and symptoms
NOTE: Information appearing in [] has been added by the authors to clarify and facilitate the use of
　　　nursing diagnoses.

ETIOLOGY

RELATED FACTORS: ○ Exposure to hot environment; inappropriate clothing ○ Vigorous activity; dehydration ○ Inability or decreased ability to perspire ○ Medications/anesthesia ○ Increased metabolic rate; illness or trauma

SIGNS
AND
SYMPTOMS

DEFINING CHARACTERISTICS:

SUBJECTIVE: ■ Increase in body temperature above normal range ○ [Headache]

OBJECTIVE: ○ Flushed skin, warm to touch ○ Increased respiratory rate, tachycardia ○ Seizures/convulsions ○ [Unstable blood pressure] ○ [Muscle rigidity/fasciculations] ○ [Confusion]

Hypothermia

PROBLEM

DEFINITION: The state in which an individual's body temperature is reduced below normal range.

ETIOLOGY

RELATED FACTORS: ○ Exposure to cool or cold environment, [prolonged exposure, immersion in cold water/near drowning, artificial hypothermia/cardiopulmonary bypass] ○ Inadequate clothing ○ Evaporation from skin in cool environment ○ Inability or decreased ability to shiver ○ Aging [or very young] ○ [Debilitating] illness or trauma, damage to hypothalamus ○ Malnutrition; decreased metabolic rate; inactivity ○ Consumption of alcohol; medications causing vasodilation ○ [Vasodilation, e.g., sepsis, drug overdose]

SIGNS
AND
SYMPTOMS

DEFINING CHARACTERISTICS:

OBJECTIVE: ■ Reduction in body temperature below normal range ■ Shivering (mild) ■ Cool skin ■ Pallor (moderate) ○ Slow capillary refill ○ Cyanotic nail beds ○ Hypertension; tachycardia ○ Piloerection ○ [Core temperature 95°F/35°C: decreased pulse, increased respiration, poor judgment, memory loss] ○ [Core temperature 94 to 90°F/34.4 to 32°C: all vital signs decreased, myocardial irritability/dysrhythmias, muscle rigidity, no shivering, obtunded] ○ [Core temperature 85°F/29.5°C: no apparent vital signs, heart rate unresponsive to drug therapy, cyanotic, dilated pupils, appears dead]

Incontinence, Functional

PROBLEM

DEFINITION: The state in which an individual experiences an involuntary, unpredictable passage of urine.

ETIOLOGY

RELATED FACTORS: ○ Altered environment [e.g., poor lighting or inability to locate bathroom] ○ Sensory, cognitive [e.g., inattentiveness to urge to void, use of sedation], or mobility deficits [including difficulty in removing clothes] ○ [Increased urine production] ○ [Reluctance to use call light or bedpan]

■ = critical factors/major signs and symptoms
NOTE: Information appearing in [] has been added by the authors to clarify and facilitate the use of
      nursing diagnoses.

DEFINING CHARACTERISTICS:

SUBJECTIVE: ■ Urge to void or bladder contractions sufficiently strong to result in loss of urine before reaching an appropriate receptacle ○ [Voiding in large amounts]

SIGNS AND SYMPTOMS

Incontinence, Reflex

DEFINITION: The state in which an individual experiences an involuntary loss of urine, occurring at somewhat predictable intervals when a specific bladder volume is reached.

PROBLEM

RELATED FACTORS: ○ Neurologic impairment (e.g., spinal cord lesion which interferes with conduction of cerebral messages above the level of the reflex arc) ○ [Cerebral lesion abolishing voluntary control]

ETIOLOGY

DEFINING CHARACTERISTICS:

SUBJECTIVE: ■ No [or only partial] awareness of bladder filling ■ No urge to void or feelings of bladder fullness ○ [Voids in large amounts] ○ [Unaware of being incontinent]

OBJECTIVE: ■ Uninhibited bladder contraction/spasm at regular intervals

SIGNS AND SYMPTOMS

Incontinence, Stress

DEFINITION: The state in which an individual experiences a loss of urine of less than 50 ml occurring with increased abdominal pressure.

PROBLEM

RELATED FACTORS: ○ Degenerative changes in pelvic muscles and structural supports associated with increased age; high intra-abdominal pressure (e.g., obesity, gravid uterus); incompetent bladder outlet; overdistention between voidings; weak pelvic muscles and structural supports

ETIOLOGY

DEFINING CHARACTERISTICS:

SUBJECTIVE: ■ Reported (or observed) dribbling with increased abdominal pressure [e.g., coughing, sneezing, lifting, impact aerobics, changing position] ○ Urinary urgency/frequency (more often than every 2 hours)

SIGNS AND SYMPTOMS

Incontinence, Total

DEFINITION: The state in which an individual experiences a continuous and unpredictable loss of urine.

PROBLEM

RELATED FACTORS: ○ Neuropathy preventing transmission of reflex [signals to the reflex arc] indicating bladder fullness ○ Neurologic dysfunction causing triggering of micturition at unpredictable times [cerebral lesions] ○ Independent contraction of detrusor reflex due to surgery ○ Trauma or disease affect-

ETIOLOGY

■ = critical factors/major signs and symptoms
NOTE: Information appearing in [] has been added by the authors to clarify and facilitate the use of nursing diagnoses.

ing spinal cord nerves [destruction of sensory or motor neurons below the spinal cord level] ○ Anatomic (fistula)

SIGNS
AND
SYMPTOMS

DEFINING CHARACTERISTICS:

SUBJECTIVE: ■ Constant flow of urine occurs at unpredictable times without distention or uninhibited bladder contractions/spasm ■ Nocturia ○ Lack of perineal or bladder filling awareness ○ Unawareness of incontinence

OBJECTIVE: ■ Unsuccessful incontinence refractory treatments

Incontinence, Urge

PROBLEM

DEFINITION: The state in which an individual experiences involuntary passage of urine occurring soon after a strong sense of urgency to void.

ETIOLOGY

RELATED FACTORS: ○ Decreased bladder capacity (e.g., history of PID, abdominal surgeries, indwelling urinary catheter) ○ Irritation of bladder stretch receptors causing spasm (e.g., bladder infection); alcohol; caffeine; increased fluids; increased urine concentration; overdistention of bladder

SIGNS
AND
SYMPTOMS

DEFINING CHARACTERISTICS:

SUBJECTIVE: ■ Urinary urgency ■ Frequency (voiding more often than every 2 hours) ■ Bladder contracture/spasm ○ Nocturia (more than two times per night)

OBJECTIVE: ○ Inability to reach toilet in time ○ Voiding in small amounts (less than 100 ml) or in large amounts (more than 550 ml)

Infection, high risk for*

PROBLEM

DEFINITION: The state in which an individual is at increased risk for being invaded by pathogenic organisms.

ETIOLOGY

RISK FACTORS: ○ Inadequate primary defenses (broken skin, traumatized tissue, decrease in ciliary action, stasis of body fluids, change in pH secretions, altered peristalsis) ○ Inadequate secondary defenses (e.g., decreased hemoglobin, leukopenia, suppressed inflammatory response) and immunosuppression ○ Inadequate acquired immunity; tissue destruction and increased environmental exposure ○ Chronic disease; malnutrition; trauma ○ Invasive procedures ○ Pharmaceutical agents ○ Rupture of amniotic membranes ○ Insufficient knowledge to avoid exposure to pathogens

---

■ = critical factors/major signs and symptoms
NOTE: Information appearing in [] has been added by the authors to clarify and facilitate the use of nursing diagnoses.
***[NOTE:** A high risk diagnosis is *not* evidenced by signs and symptoms, since the problem has not yet occurred, and nursing interventions are directed at prevention. Therefore, risk factors which are present are noted instead.]

Injury, high risk for*

DEFINITION: A state in which the individual is at risk of injury as a result of environmental conditions interacting with the individual's adaptive and defensive resources. [*Note:* The potential for injury differs from individual to individual and situation to situation. It is our belief that the environment is not safe, and there is no way to list everything that might present a danger to someone. Rather, we believe nurses have the responsibility to educate people throughout their life cycles to live safely in their environment.]

PROBLEM

RISK FACTORS:

ETIOLOGY

INTERNAL: ○ Biochemical, regulatory function: (sensory, integrative, effector dysfunction; tissue hypoxia), immune-autoimmune; malnutrition; abnormal blood profile, (leukocytosis/leukopenia; altered clotting factors; thrombocytopenia; sickle cell, thalassemia; decreased hemoglobin) ○ Physical: (broken skin, altered mobility); development age; (physiologic, psychosocial) ○ Psychologic: (affective, orientation)

EXTERNAL: ○ Biologic, (immunization level of community, microorganism) ○ Chemical: (pollutants, poisons, drugs, pharmaceutical agents, alcohol, caffeine, nicotine, preservatives, cosmetics, and dyes), nutrients (vitamins, food types) ○ Physical: (design, structure, and arrangement of community, building, and/or equipment); mode of transport/transportation ○ People-provider: (nosocomial agent; staffing patterns; cognitive, affective, and psychomotor factors)

Knowledge Deficit (specify) [Learning Need]

DEFINITION: [Lack of specific information necessary for patient/significant other(s) to make informed choices regarding condition/therapies/treatment plan.]

PROBLEM

RELATED FACTORS: ○ Lack of exposure ○ Information misinterpretation ○ Unfamiliarity with information resources ○ Lack of recall ○ Cognitive limitation ○ Lack of interest in learning ○ [Patient's request for no information] ○ [Inaccurate/incomplete information presented]

ETIOLOGY

DEFINING CHARACTERISTICS:

SIGNS
AND
SYMPTOMS

SUBJECTIVE: ○ Verbalization of the problem ○ [Request for information] ○ [Statement of misconception]

OBJECTIVE: ○ Inaccurate follow-through of instruction ○ Inadequate performance of test ○ Inappropriate or exaggerated behaviors, for example, hysterical, hostile, agitated, apathetic ○ [Development of preventable complication]

■ = critical factors/major signs and symptoms
NOTE: Information appearing in [] has been added by the authors to clarify and facilitate the use of nursing diagnoses.
*[NOTE: A high risk diagnosis is *not* evidenced by signs and symptoms, since the problem has not yet occurred, and nursing interventions are directed at prevention. Therefore, risk factors which are present are noted instead.]

Noncompliance [Compliance, altered] (specify)

PROBLEM

DEFINITION: A person's informed decision not to adhere to a therapeutic recommendation. [*Note: Noncompliance* is a term that may create a negative situation for patient and caregiver that may foster difficulties in resolving the causative factors. Since patients have a right to refuse therapy, we see this as a situation in which the professional need is to accept the patient's point of view/behavior/choice(s) and work together to find alternate means to meet original and/or revised goals.]

ETIOLOGY

RELATED FACTORS: ○ Patient value system: health beliefs, cultural influences, spiritual values ○ Client–provider relationships ○ [Fear/Anxiety]

SIGNS
AND
SYMPTOMS

DEFINING CHARACTERISTICS:

SUBJECTIVE: ■ Statements by patient or significant other(s), [e.g., unwillingness to follow treatment regimen]

OBJECTIVE: ■ Behavior indicative of failure to adhere (by direct observation) ○ Objective tests (physiologic measures, detection of markers) ○ Failure to progress ○ Evidence of development of complications; exacerbation of symptoms ○ Failure to keep appointments ○ [Inability to set or attain mutual goals]

Nutrition, altered: high risk for more than body requirements*

PROBLEM

DEFINITION: The state in which an individual is at risk of experiencing an intake of nutrients which exceeds metabolic needs.

ETIOLOGY

RISK FACTORS: ■ Reported/observed obesity in one or both parents[/spouse; hereditary predisposition] ■ Rapid transition across growth percentiles in infants or children, [adolescence] ○ Reported use of solid food as major food source before 5 months of age ○ Reported/observed higher base-line weight at beginning of each pregnancy ○ Dysfunctional eating patterns:

Pairing food with other activities;
Eating in response to external cues such as time of day or social situation;
Concentrating food intake at end of day;
Eating in response to internal cues other than hunger, for example, anxiety

○ Observed use of food as reward or comfort measure ○ [Socially/culturally isolated; lacking other outlets] ○ [Alteration in usual activity patterns/sedentary lifestyle] ○ [Alteration in usual coping patterns] ○ [Majority of foods consumed are concentrated, high-calorie sources] ○ [Significant/sudden decline in financial resources, lower socioeconomic status]

■ = critical factors/major signs and symptoms
NOTE: Information appearing in [] has been added by the authors to clarify and facilitate the use of nursing diagnoses.

*[NOTE: A high risk diagnosis is *not* evidenced by signs and symptoms, since the problem has not yet occurred, and nursing interventions are directed at prevention. Therefore, risk factors which are present are noted instead.]

Nutrition, altered, less than body requirements

DEFINITION: The state in which an individual experiences an intake of nutrients insufficient to meet metabolic needs.

PROBLEM

RELATED FACTORS: ○ Inability to ingest or digest food or absorb nutrients due to biologic, psychologic, or economic factors ○ [Intake insufficient to meet metabolic demands]

ETIOLOGY

DEFINING CHARACTERISTICS:

SIGNS
AND
SYMPTOMS

SUBJECTIVE: ○ Reported inadequate food intake less than RDA ○ Reported or evidence of lack of food ○ Aversion to eating ○ Reported altered taste sensation ○ Abdominal pain with or without pathologic conditions ○ Lack of interest in food ○ Perceived inability to ingest food ○ Satiety immediately after ingesting food ○ Abdominal cramping ○ Lack of information, misinformation, misconceptions

OBJECTIVE: ○ Body weight 20 percent or more under ideal [for height and frame] ○ Loss of weight with adequate food intake ○ Poor muscle tone ○ Weakness of muscles required for swallowing or mastication ○ Sore, inflamed buccal cavity ○ Capillary fragility ○ Hyperactive bowel sounds ○ Diarrhea and/or steatorrhea ○ Pale conjunctiva and mucous membranes ○ Excessive loss of hair [or increased growth of hair on body (lanugo)] ○ [Decreased subcutaneous fat/muscle mass] ○ [Cessation of menses]

Nutrition, altered, more than body requirements

DEFINITION: The state in which an individual is experiencing an intake of nutrients which exceeds metabolic needs.

PROBLEM

RELATED FACTORS: ○ Excessive intake in relationship to metabolic need
Note: Underlying cause is often complex and may be difficult to diagnose/ treat.

ETIOLOGY

DEFINING CHARACTERISTICS:

SIGNS
AND
SYMPTOMS

SUBJECTIVE: ○ Reported dysfunctional eating patterns:
Pairing food with other activities;
Eating in response to external cues such as time of day, social situation;
Concentrating food intake at end of day;
Eating in response to internal cues other than hunger, for example, anxiety
○ Sedentary activity level

OBJECTIVE: ■ Weight 20 percent over ideal for height and frame ■ Triceps skin fold greater than 15 mm in men and 25 mm in women ○ Weight 10 percent over ideal for height and frame ○ Observed dysfunctional eating pat-

---

■ = critical factors/major signs and symptoms
NOTE: Information appearing in [] has been added by the authors to clarify and facilitate the use of nursing diagnoses.

terns [as noted in Subjective] ○ [Percentage of body fat greater than: 18–20 percent for trim women; 10–12 percent for trim men.]

Oral Mucous Membrane, altered

PROBLEM

DEFINITION: The state in which the individual experiences disruptions in the tissue layers of the oral cavity.

ETIOLOGY

RELATED FACTORS: ○ Pathologic conditions: oral cavity (radiation to head and/or neck) ○ Trauma:

> Chemical, for example, acidic foods, drugs, noxious agents, alcohol; Mechanical, for example, ill-fitting dentures, braces, tubes (endotracheal, naso-gastric), surgery (in oral cavity)

○ Dehydration; malnutrition ○ NPO for more than 24 hours ○ Lack of or decreased salivation ○ Ineffective oral hygiene; infection ○ Mouth breathing ○ Medication

SIGNS
AND
SYMPTOMS

DEFINING CHARACTERISTICS:

> **SUBJECTIVE:** ○ Xerostomia (dry mouth) ○ Oral pain/discomfort

> **OBJECTIVE:** ○ Lack of or decreased salivation ○ Coated tongue ○ Stomatitis; leukoplakia; hyperemia ○ Hemorrhagic gingivitis; vesicles ○ Halitosis; carious teeth ○ Oral lesions or ulcers; desquamation ○ Edema ○ Oral plaque

Pain [acute]

PROBLEM

DEFINITION: A state in which an individual experiences and reports the presence of severe discomfort or an uncomfortable sensation.

ETIOLOGY

RELATED FACTORS: ○ Injuring agents (biologic, chemical, physical, psychologic)

SIGNS
AND
SYMPTOMS

DEFINING CHARACTERISTICS:

> **SUBJECTIVE:** ○ Communication (verbal or coded) of pain descriptors

> [Expect less from under age 40, males, and some cultural groups]

○ [Pain unrelieved and/or increased beyond tolerance]

> **OBJECTIVE:** ○ Distraction behavior (moaning, crying, pacing, seeking out other people and/or activities, restlessness) ○ Guarding behavior, protective ○ Alteration in muscle tone (may span from listless to rigid) ○ Facial mask of pain (eyes lack luster, "beaten look," fixed or scattered movement, grimace) ○ Autonomic responses not seen in chronic, stable pain (diaphoresis, blood pressure and pulse change, pupillary dilation, increased or decreased respiratory rate) ○ Self-focusing ○ Narrowed focus (altered time perception, withdrawal from social contact, impaired thought process) ○ [Fear/panic]

■ = critical factors/major signs and symptoms
NOTE: Information appearing in [] has been added by the authors to clarify and facilitate the use of nursing diagnoses.

Pain, chronic

DEFINITION: A state in which the individual experiences pain that continues for more than 6 months. [Pain is a signal that something is wrong, and chronic pain is a learned form of behavior. It is a complex, separate entity, combining elements from other NDs: Powerlessness; Diversional Activity, altered; Family Processes, altered; Self-care deficit, etc.]   PROBLEM

RELATED FACTORS: ○ Chronic physical/psychosocial disability   ETIOLOGY

DEFINING CHARACTERISTICS: SIGNS AND SYMPTOMS

SUBJECTIVE: ■ Verbal report of pain experienced for more than 6 months ○ Fear of reinjury ○ Altered ability to continue previous activities ○ Anorexia, weight changes ○ Changes in sleep patterns ○ [Preoccupation with pain] ○ [Desperately seeks alternative solutions/therapies for relief/control of pain]

OBJECTIVE: ■ Observed evidence of pain experienced for more than 6 months ○ Physical and social withdrawal ○ Facial mask, guarded movement

Parental Role Conflict

DEFINITION: The state in which a parent experiences role confusion and conflict in response to crisis.   PROBLEM

RELATED FACTORS: ○ Separation from child due to chronic illness ○ Intimidation with invasive or restrictive modalities (e.g., isolation, intubation) specialized care centers, policies ○ Home care of a child with special needs (e.g., apnea monitoring, postural drainage, hyperalimentation) ○ Change in marital status ○ Interruptions of family life due to home care regimen (treatments, caregivers, lack of respite)   ETIOLOGY

DEFINING CHARACTERISTICS: SIGNS AND SYMPTOMS

SUBJECTIVE: ■ Parent(s) express concerns/feelings of inadequacy to provide for child's physical and emotional needs during hospitalization or in the home ■ Parent(s) express concerns about changes in parental role, family functioning, family communication, family health ○ Parent(s) express concern about perceived loss of control over decisions relating to their child ○ Parent(s) verbalize feelings of guilt, anger, fear, anxiety, and/or frustration about effect of child's illness on family process

OBJECTIVE: ■ Demonstrated disruption in care taking routines ○ Reluctance to participate in usual care taking activities even with encouragement and support ○ Demonstrated feelings of guilt, anger, fear, anxiety, and/or frustration about effect of child's illness on family process

---

■ = critical factors/major signs and symptoms
NOTE: Information appearing in [] has been added by the authors to clarify and facilitate the use of nursing diagnoses.

Parenting, altered

PROBLEM

DEFINITION: The state in which a nurturing figure(s) experiences an inability to create an environment which promotes the optimum growth and development of another human being. (It is important to state as a preface to this diagnosis that adjustment to parenting in general is a normal maturational process that elicits nursing behaviors of prevention of potential problems and health promotion.)

ETIOLOGY

RELATED FACTORS: ○ Lack of available role model; ineffective role model ○ Lack of support between/from significant other(s) ○ Interruption in bonding process, that is, maternal, paternal, other ○ Mental and/or physical illness ○ Lack of knowledge ○ Limited cognitive functioning ○ Multiple pregnancies ○ Unrealistic expectation for self, infant, partner ○ Physical and psychosocial abuse of nurturing figure ○ Unmet social/emotional maturation needs of parenting figures ○ Perceived threat to own survival, physical and emotional ○ Presence of stress (financial, legal, recent crisis, cultural move [e.g., from another country, nationality]) ○ Lack of role identity ○ Lack of appropriate response of child to relationship

SIGNS
AND
SYMPTOMS

DEFINING CHARACTERISTICS:

SUBJECTIVE: ■ Verbalization cannot control child ○ Constant verbalization of disappointment in gender or physical characteristics of the infant/child ○ Verbalization of resentment toward the infant/child ○ Verbalization of role inadequacy [inability to care for/discipline child] ○ Verbal disgust at body functions of infant/child ○ Verbalizes desire to have child call him/herself by first name versus traditional cultural tendencies

OBJECTIVE: ■ Abandonment; runaway ■ Incidence of physical and psychologic trauma ■ Inattention to infant/child needs ■ Inappropriate care taking behaviors (toilet training, sleep/rest, feeding) ■ History of child abuse or abandonment by primary caretaker ○ Lack of parental attachment behaviors:

Inappropriate visual, tactile, auditory stimulation;
Negative identification of infant/child characteristics;
Negative attachment of meanings to infant/child characteristics;
Noncompliance with health appointments for self and/or infant/child

○ Inappropriate or inconsistent discipline practices ○ Frequent accidents/illness ○ Growth and development lag in the child ○ Child receives care from multiple caretakers without consideration for the needs of the infant/child ○ Compulsive seeking of role approval from others

---

■ = critical factors/major signs and symptoms
NOTE: Information appearing in [] has been added by the authors to clarify and facilitate the use of nursing diagnoses.

Parenting, altered, high risk*

DEFINITION: The state in which a nurturing figure(s) is at risk to experience an inability to create an environment which promotes the optimum growth and development of another human being. (It is important to state as a preface to this diagnosis that adjustment to parenting in general is a normal maturational process that elicits nursing behaviors of prevention of potential problems and health promotion.) PROBLEM

RISK FACTORS:† ○ Lack of available role model; ineffective role model ○ Lack of support between/from significant other(s) ○ Interruption in bonding process, that is, maternal, paternal, other ○ Mental and/or physical illness ○ Lack of knowledge ○ Limited cognitive functioning ○ Multiple pregnancies ○ Unrealistic expectation for self, infant, partner ○ Physical and psychosocial abuse of nurturing figure ○ Unmet social/emotional maturation needs of parenting figures ○ Perceived threat to own survival, physical and emotional ○ Presence of stress (financial, legal, recent crisis, cultural move [e.g., from another country, nationality]) ○ Lack of role identity ○ Lack of appropriate response of child to relationship ETIOLOGY

Personal Identity, disturbance

DEFINITION: Inability to distinguish between self and nonself. PROBLEM

RELATED FACTORS: ○ To be developed by NANDA ○ [Organic brain syndrome] ○ [Poor ego differentiation, as in Schizophrenia] ○ [Panic/dissociative states] ○ [Biochemical body change] ETIOLOGY

DEFINING CHARACTERISTICS: ○ To be developed by NANDA SIGNS AND SYMPTOMS

 SUBJECTIVE: ○ [Confusion about sense of self, purpose or direction in life, sexual identification/preference]

 OBJECTIVE: ○ [Difficulty in making decisions] ○ [Poorly differentiated ego boundaries] ○ [See ND Anxiety, Panic State]

Physical Mobility, impaired [specify, level]

DEFINITION: A state in which the individual experiences a limitation of ability for independent physical movement. PROBLEM

RELATED FACTORS: ○ Intolerance to activity/decreased strength and endurance ○ Pain/discomfort ○ Neuromuscular/musculoskeletal impairment ○ ETIOLOGY

■ = critical factors/major signs and symptoms

NOTE: Information appearing in [] has been added by the authors to clarify and facilitate the use of nursing diagnoses.

*[NOTE: A high risk diagnosis is *not* evidenced by signs and symptoms, since the problem has not yet occurred, and nursing interventions are directed at prevention. Therefore, risk factors which are present are noted instead.]

† NANDA has currently identified these as Related Factors. However, we believe they are Risk Factors. We believe that the presence of the "Risk Factors" originally identified by NANDA would indicate an actual problem.

Perceptual/cognitive impairment ○ Depression/severe anxiety ○ [Restrictive therapies/safety precautions, e.g., bed rest, limb immobilization]

SIGNS
AND
SYMPTOMS

DEFINING CHARACTERISTICS:

SUBJECTIVE: ○ Reluctance to attempt movement ○ [Complaints of pain/discomfort on movement]

OBJECTIVE: ○ Inability to purposefully move within the physical environment, including bed mobility, transfer, and ambulation ○ Impaired coordination ○ Limited range of motion ○ Decreased muscle strength, control, and/or mass ○ Imposed restrictions of movement, including mechanical, medical protocol

Suggested Functional Level Classification:

0 = Completely independent;
1 = Requires use of equipment or device;
2 = Requires help from another person for assistance, supervision, or teaching;
3 = Requires help from another person and equipment device;
4 = Dependent, does not participate in activity (Code adapted from E. Jones, et al., Patient Classification for Long-term Care: User's Manual, HEW, Publication No. HRA-74-3107, November 1974.)

Poisoning, high risk for*

PROBLEM

DEFINITION: Accentuated risk of accidental exposure to or ingestion of drugs or dangerous products in dosages sufficient to cause poisoning.

ETIOLOGY

RISK FACTORS

INTERNAL (INDIVIDUAL): ○ Reduced vision ○ Lack of safety or drug education ○ Lack of proper precaution ○ Insufficient finances ○ Verbalization of occupational setting without adequate safeguards ○ Cognitive or emotional difficulties

EXTERNAL (ENVIRONMENTAL): ○ Large supplies of drugs in house ○ Dangerous products placed or stored within the reach of children or confused persons ○ Flaking, peeling paint or plaster in presence of young children ○ Paint, lacquer, and so on, in poorly ventilated areas or without effective protection ○ Medicines stored in unlocked cabinets accessible to children or confused persons ○ Availability of illicit drugs potentially contaminated by poisonous additives ○ Chemical contamination of food and water ○ Unprotected contact with heavy metals or chemicals ○ Presence of poisonous vegetation ○ Presence of atmospheric pollutants

---

■ = critical factors/major signs and symptoms

NOTE: Information appearing in [] has been added by the authors to clarify and facilitate the use of nursing diagnoses.

***[NOTE:** A high risk diagnosis is *not* evidenced by signs and symptoms, since the problem has not yet occurred, and nursing interventions are directed at prevention. Therefore, risk factors which are present are noted instead.]

Post-Trauma Response [specify stage]

DEFINITION: The state of an individual's experiencing a sustained painful response to an overwhelming traumatic event.

PROBLEM

RELATED FACTORS: ○ Disasters [e.g., floods, earthquakes, tornadoes, airplane crashes], wars, epidemics, rape, assault, torture, catastrophic illness, or accident, [being held hostage].

ETIOLOGY

DEFINING CHARACTERISTICS

SIGNS
AND
SYMPTOMS

SUBJECTIVE: ■ Reexperience of the traumatic event which may be identified in cognitive, affective, and/or sensory motor activities (flashbacks, intrusive thoughts, repetitive dreams or nightmares, excessive verbalization of the traumatic event, verbalization of survival guilt or guilt about behavior required for survival) ○ [Somatic reactions: chronic pains, nausea, changes in appetite, skeletal/muscle tension, exaggerated startle response, sensitivity to noise, insomnia, headaches, dizziness, unsteadiness, chronic fatigue and easy fatigability, sleep disturbance]

OBJECTIVE: ○ Psychic/emotional numbness (impaired interpretation of reality, confusion, dissociation or amnesia, vagueness about traumatic event, constricted affect) ○ Altered lifestyle (self-destructiveness such as substance abuse, suicide attempt or other acting out behavior, difficulty with interpersonal relationships, [loss of interest in usual activities, detachment, loss of feeling of intimacy/sexuality], development of phobia regarding trauma, poor impulse control/irritability and explosiveness) ○ [Disturbance of mood, e.g., depression, anxiety, embarrassment, fear, humiliation, self-blame, low self-esteem, fear of violence toward self or others] ○ [Cognitive disruption: confusion, loss of memory/concentration, indecisiveness] ○ [Social reactions: dependence on others, work/school failure, avoidance of close relationships, social isolation]

[Stages:

Acute Subtype: begins within 6 months and does not last longer than 6 months;

Chronic subtype: lasts more than 6 months;

Delayed subtype: period of latency of 6 months or more before onset of symptoms]

Powerlessness [specify level]

DEFINITION: Perception that one's own action will not significantly affect an outcome; a perceived lack of control over a current situation or immediate happening.

PROBLEM

RELATED FACTORS: ○ Healthcare environment ○ Interpersonal interaction ○ Illness-related regimen ○ Lifestyle of helplessness

ETIOLOGY

■ = critical factors/major signs and symptoms
NOTE: Information appearing in [] has been added by the authors to clarify and facilitate the use of nursing diagnoses.

SIGNS
AND
SYMPTOMS

DEFINING CHARACTERISTICS

    SUBJECTIVE

Severe:

○ Verbal expressions of having no control or influence over situation, outcome, or self-care ○ Depression over physical deterioration which occurs despite patient compliance with regimens

Moderate:

○ Nonparticipation in care or decision-making when opportunities are provided ○ Expressions of dissatisfaction and frustration over inability to perform previous tasks and/or activities ○ Expression of doubt regarding role performance ○ Reluctance to express true feelings; fearing alienation from caregivers

Low:

○ Expressions of uncertainty about fluctuating energy levels

    OBJECTIVE

Severe:

○ Apathy; [withdrawn, resigned, crying] ○ [Anger]

Moderate:

○ Does not monitor progress ○ Dependence on others that may result in irritability, resentment, anger, and guilt ○ Inability to seek information regarding care ○ Does not defend self-care practices when challenged ○ Passivity

Low:

○ Passivity

Protection, altered

PROBLEM

DEFINITION: The state in which an individual experiences a decrease in the ability to guard the self from internal or external threats such as illness or injury.

ETIOLOGY

RELATED FACTORS: ○ Extremes of age ○ Inadequate nutrition ○ Alcohol abuse ○ Abnormal blood profiles (leukopenia, thrombocytopenia, anemia, coagulation) ○ Drug therapies (antineoplastic, corticosteroid, immune, anticoagulant, thrombolytic) ○ Treatments (surgery, radiation) ○ Diseases (such as cancer and immune disorders)

SIGNS
AND
SYMPTOMS

DEFINING CHARACTERISTICS

    SUBJECTIVE: ■ Neurosensory alterations ○ Chilling ○ Itching ○ Insomnia; fatigue; weakness ○ Anorexia

    OBJECTIVE: ■ Deficient immunity ■ Impaired healing ■ Altered clotting ■ Maladaptive stress response ○ Perspiring ○ Dyspnea; cough ○ Restlessness; immobility ○ Disorientation ○ Pressure sores

---

■ = critical factors/major signs and symptoms

NOTE: Information appearing in [] has been added by the authors to clarify and facilitate the use of nursing diagnoses.

[*Note:* The purpose of this diagnosis seems to be to provide for the combining of multiple diagnoses under a single heading for ease of planning care when a number of variables may be present.]

Rape-Trauma Syndrome [specify]

DEFINITION: Forced, violent sexual penetration against the victim's will and consent. The trauma syndrome that develops from this attack or attempted attack includes an acute phase of disorganization of the victim's lifestyle and a long-term process of reorganization of lifestyle. (This syndrome includes the following three subcomponents: Rape trauma compound (A); Compound reaction (B), and Silent reaction (C). [*Note:* While attacks are most often directed toward women, men also may be victims.]

PROBLEM

DEFINING CHARACTERISTICS

SIGNS
AND
SYMPTOMS

A: RAPE TRAUMA

Acute Phase:

○ Emotional reactions (anger, embarrassment, fear of physical violence and death, humiliation, revenge, self-blame) ○ Multiple physical symptoms (gastrointestinal irritability, genitourinary discomfort, muscle tension, sleep pattern disturbance)

Long-Term Phase:

○ Changes in lifestyle (change in residence; dealing with repetitive nightmares and phobias; seeking family support; seeking social network support)

B: COMPOUND REACTION: All defining characteristics listed under rape trauma; in addition: ○ Reactivated symptoms of such previous conditions, that is, physical/psychiatric illness ○ Reliance on alcohol and/or drugs

C: SILENT REACTION: ○ Abrupt changes in relationships with men ○ Increase in nightmares ○ Increasing anxiety during interview, that is, blocking of associations, long periods of silence, minor stuttering, physical distress ○ Pronounced changes in sexual behavior ○ No verbalization of the occurrence of rape ○ Sudden onset of phobic reactions

Role Performance, altered

DEFINITION: Disruption in the way one perceives one's role performance.

PROBLEM

RELATED FACTORS: ○ To be developed by NANDA ○ [Crisis:]

ETIOLOGY

[Situational, e.g., male head of the household is in a passive, dependent patient role];
[Developmental]; and/or
[Health-illness, e.g., chronic illness]

■ = critical factors/major signs and symptoms
NOTE: Information appearing in [] has been added by the authors to clarify and facilitate the use of nursing diagnoses.

SIGNS
AND
SYMPTOMS

DEFINING CHARACTERISTICS

SUBJECTIVE: ○ Change in self-perception of role ○ Denial of role ○ Lack of knowledge of role

OBJECTIVE: ○ Change in others' perception of role ○ Change in usual patterns or responsibility ○ Conflict in roles ○ Change in physical capacity to resume role ○ [Failure to assume role]

Self-Care Deficit: feeding, bathing/hygiene, dressing/grooming, toileting

PROBLEM

DEFINITION: A state in which the individual experiences an impaired ability to perform or complete feeding, bathing/hygiene, dressing/grooming, or toileting activities for oneself [on a temporary, permanent, or progressing basis]. [*Note:* Self-Care may also be expanded to include the practices used by the patient to promote health, the individual responsibility for self, a way of thinking. Refer to Home Maintenance Management, impaired; Health Maintenance, altered.]

ETIOLOGY

RELATED FACTORS: ○ Intolerance to activity; decreased strength and endurance ○ Neuromuscular/musculoskeletal impairment ○ Depression; severe anxiety ○ Pain, discomfort ○ Perceptual or cognitive impairment

SIGNS
AND
SYMPTOMS

DEFINING CHARACTERISTICS

a. Self-Feeding deficit (levels 0 to 4)†
   ○ Inability to bring food from a receptacle to the mouth
b. Self-Bathing/Hygiene deficit (levels 0 to 4)†
   ■ Inability to wash body or body parts ■ Inability to obtain or get to water source; regulate temperature or flow
c. Self-Dressing/Grooming deficit (levels 0 to 4)†
   ○ Impaired ability to put on or take off necessary items of clothing; obtain or replace articles of clothing; fasten clothing; maintain appearance at a satisfactory level
d. Self-toileting deficit (levels 0 to 4)†

   Related Factors (in addition to those previously noted): ○ Impaired transfer ability ○ Intolerance to activity; decreased strength and endurance ○ Impaired mobility status
   Defining Characteristics: (Objective) ■ Unable to get to toilet or commode ■ Unable to manipulate clothing for toileting ■ Unable to sit on or rise from toilet or commode ■ Unable to carry out proper toilet hygiene ○ Unable to flush toilet or empty commode

---

■ = critical factors/major signs and symptoms
NOTE: Information appearing in [] has been added by the authors to clarify and facilitate the use of nursing diagnoses.
† Refer to ND Physical Mobility, impaired, for definition of levels.

Self-Esteem, Chronic Low

DEFINITION: Longstanding negative self-evaluation/feelings about self or self-capabilities

PROBLEM

RELATED FACTORS: ○ [Continual negative evaluation of self/capabilities during childhood] ○ [Personal vulnerability] ○ [Life choices perpetuating failure]

ETIOLOGY

DEFINING CHARACTERISTICS

SIGNS AND SYMPTOMS

SUBJECTIVE: Longstanding or chronic: ■ Self-negating verbalization ■ Expressions of shame/guilt ■ Evaluates self as unable to deal with events ■ Rationalizes away/rejects positive feedback and exaggerates negative feedback about self

OBJECTIVE: ■ Hesitant to try new things/situations ○ Frequent lack of success in work or other life events ○ Overly conforming, dependent on others' opinions ○ Lack of eye contact ○ Nonassertive/passive; indecisive ○ Excessively seeks reassurance

Self-Esteem disturbance

DEFINITION: Negative self-evaluation/feelings about self or self-capabilities which may be directly or indirectly expressed. [A human need for survival.]

PROBLEM

RELATED FACTORS: ○ ["Failure" at life events, e.g., loss of job, divorce] ○ [Aging]

ETIOLOGY

DEFINING CHARACTERISTICS

SIGNS AND SYMPTOMS

SUBJECTIVE: ○ Self-negating verbalization ○ Evaluates self as unable to deal with events ○ Expressions of shame/guilt ○ Rationalizes away/rejects positive feedback and exaggerates negative feedback about self ○ [Inability to accept positive reinforcement]

OBJECTIVE: ○ Hesitant to try new things/situations ○ Hypersensitive to slight or criticism ○ Grandiosity ○ Denial of problems obvious to others ○ Projection of blame/responsibility for problems ○ Rationalizing personal failures ○ [Not taking responsibility for self-care (self-neglect)] ○ [Lack of follow-through] ○ [Nonparticipation in therapy] ○ [Self-destructive behavior] ○ [Lack of eye contact]

Self-Esteem, Situational Low

DEFINITION: Negative self-evaluation/feelings about self which develop in response to a loss or change in an individual who previously had a positive self-evaluation.

PROBLEM

RELATED FACTORS: ○ ["Failure" at life events, e.g., loss of job, divorce] ○ [Aging]

ETIOLOGY

■ = critical factors/major signs and symptoms
NOTE: Information appearing in [] has been added by the authors to clarify and facilitate the use of nursing diagnoses.

SIGNS
AND
SYMPTOMS

DEFINING CHARACTERISTICS

SUBJECTIVE: ■ Episodic occurrence of negative self-appraisal in response to life events in a person with a previous positive self-evaluation ■ Verbalization of negative feelings about the self (helplessness, uselessness) ○ Self-negating verbalizations; expressions of shame/guilt ○ Evaluates self as unable to handle situations/events

OBJECTIVE: ○ Difficulty making decisions

Sensory-Perceptual alterations (specify): visual, auditory, kinesthetic, gustatory, tactile, olfactory

PROBLEM

DEFINITION: A state in which an individual experiences a change in the amount or patterning of incoming stimuli accompanied by a diminished, exaggerated, distorted, or impaired response to such stimuli.

ETIOLOGY

RELATED FACTORS: ○ Altered environmental stimuli, excessive or insufficient ○ [Therapeutically restricted environments, e.g., isolation, intensive care, bed rest, traction, confining illnesses, incubator] ○ [Socially restricted environment (e.g., institutionalization, homebound, aging, chronic illness, dying, infant deprivation); stigmatized (e.g., mentally ill/retarded/handicapped); bereaved] ○ [Excessive noise level, e.g., work environment, patient's immediate environment (ICU with support machinery, etc.)] ○ Altered sensory reception, transmission, and/or integration:

> Neurologic disease, trauma, or deficit;
> Altered status of sense organs;
> Inability to communicate, understand, speak, or respond;
> Sleep deprivation; and/or
> Pain, [phantom limb]

○ Chemical alterations:

> Endogenous (electrolyte), [elevated BUN, elevated ammonia, hypoxia]; and/or
> Exogenous (drugs, etc.) [central nervous system stimulants or depressants, mind-altering drugs]

○ Psychologic stress [narrowed perceptual fields caused by anxiety]

SIGNS
AND
SYMPTOMS

DEFINING CHARACTERISTICS

SUBJECTIVE: ○ Anxiety [panic state] ○ Indication of body image alteration ○ Reported change in sensory acuity [e.g., photosensitivity, hypo/hyperesthesias, diminished/altered sense of taste, inability to tell position of body parts, proprioception] ○ [Pain]

OBJECTIVE: ○ Measured change in sensory acuity ○ Change in problem-solving abilities, [lack of/poor concentration] ○ Altered abstraction/conceptualization, [disordered thought sequencing] ○ Disoriented in time, in place, or with persons ○ Altered communication patterns ○ Change in usual

---

■ = critical factors/major signs and symptoms
NOTE: Information appearing in [] has been added by the authors to clarify and facilitate the use of nursing diagnoses.

response to stimuli, [rapid mood swings, exaggerated emotional responses] ○ Change in behavior pattern ○ Apathy ○ Restlessness, irritability ○ [Bizarre thinking] ○ [Motor incordination; altered sense of balance, e.g., Menieres' syndrome] ○ Other possible defining characteristics:

Complaints of fatigue;
Change in muscular tension;
Hallucinations;
Alteration in posture; and/or
Inappropriate responses

Sexual Dysfunction

DEFINITION: The state in which an individual experiences a change in sexual function that is viewed as unsatisfying, unrewarding, or inadequate.

PROBLEM

RELATED FACTORS: ○ Biopsychosocial alteration of sexuality:

ETIOLOGY

Ineffectual or absent role models;
Vulnerability;
Misinformation or lack of knowledge;
Physical abuse;
Values conflict;
Lack of privacy;
Altered body structure or function (pregnancy, recent childbirth, drugs, surgery, anomalies, disease process, trauma, radiation, [loss of sexual desire, disruption of sexual response pattern, e.g., premature ejaculation, dyspareunia]);
Psychosocial abuse, for example, harmful relationships; and/or
Lack of significant other

DEFINING CHARACTERISTICS

SIGNS
AND
SYMPTOMS

SUBJECTIVE: ○ Verbalization of problem ○ Actual or perceived limitation imposed by disease and/or therapy ○ Inability to achieve desired satisfaction ○ Alterations in achieving perceived sex role ○ Conflicts involving values ○ Alterations in achieving sexual satisfaction ○ Seeking of confirmation of desirability

OBJECTIVE: ○ Alteration in relationship with significant other ○ Change of interest in self and others

Sexuality Patterns, altered

DEFINITION: The state in which an individual expresses concern regarding his/her sexuality.

PROBLEM

RELATED FACTORS: ○ Knowledge/skill deficit about alternative responses to health-related transitions, altered body function or structure, illness or medi-

ETIOLOGY

■ = critical factors/major signs and symptoms
NOTE: Information appearing in [] has been added by the authors to clarify and facilitate the use of nursing diagnoses.

cal treatment ○ Lack of privacy ○ Lack of significant other ○ Ineffective or absent role models ○ Conflicts with sexual orientation or variant preferences ○ Fear of pregnancy or of acquiring a sexually transmitted disease ○ Impaired relationship with a significant other

SIGNS
AND
SYMPTOMS

DEFINING CHARACTERISTICS

SUBJECTIVE: ■ Reported difficulties, limitations, or changes in sexual behaviors or activities.

Skin Integrity, impaired

PROBLEM

DEFINITION: A state in which the individual's skin is adversely altered. [An interruption in the integumentary system, the largest, multifunctional organ of the body.]

ETIOLOGY

RELATED FACTORS:

EXTERNAL (ENVIRONMENTAL): ○ Hyperthermia or hypothermia ○ Chemical substance ○ Radiation ○ Physical immobilization ○ Humidity ○ Mechanical factors (shearing forces, pressure, restraint) ○ [Excretions/secretions] ○ [Trauma: injury/surgery]

INTERNAL (SOMATIC): ○ Medication ○ Altered nutritional state (obesity, emaciation); metabolic state; circulation; sensation; pigmentation ○ Skeletal prominence ○ Developmental factors ○ Alterations in turgor (change in elasticity) ○ Immunologic deficit ○ [Excretions/secretions] ○ [Psychogenic] ○ [Presence of edema]

SIGNS
AND
SYMPTOMS

DEFINING CHARACTERISTICS

SUBJECTIVE: ○ [Complaints of itching, pain, numbness, of affected/surrounding area]

OBJECTIVE: ○ Disruption of skin surface ○ Destruction of skin layers ○ Invasion of body structures

Skin Integrity, impaired, high risk for*

PROBLEM

DEFINITION: A state in which the individual's skin is at risk of being adversely altered.

ETIOLOGY

RISK FACTORS

EXTERNAL (ENVIRONMENTAL): ○ Chemical substance ○ Hypothermia or hyperthermia ○ Radiation ○ Physical immobilization ○ Excretions and secretions ○ Humidity ○ Mechanical factors (shearing forces, pressure, restraint)

■ = critical factors/major signs and symptoms
NOTE: Information appearing in [] has been added by the authors to clarify and facilitate the use of nursing diagnoses.
***[NOTE:** A high risk diagnosis is *not* evidenced by signs and symptoms, since the problem has not yet occurred, and nursing interventions are directed at prevention. Therefore, risk factors which are present are noted instead.]

INTERNAL (SOMATIC): ○ Medication ○ Alterations in nutrition state (obesity, emaciation); metabolic state; circulation; sensation; pigmentation ○ Skeletal prominence ○ Developmental factors ○ Alterations in skin turgor (change in elasticity) ○ Psychogenic ○ Immunologic ○ [Presence of edema]

Sleep Pattern disturbance

DEFINITION: Disruption of sleep time which causes patient discomfort or interferes with desired lifestyle.   PROBLEM

RELATED FACTORS   ETIOLOGY

SENSORY ALTERATIONS: ○ Internal (illness, [pain]; psychologic stress [anxiety, depression]; [inactivity]) ○ External (environment changes [including change of work shift, hospital routine]; social cues [e.g., demands of caring for others])

DEFINING CHARACTERISTICS   SIGNS
AND
SYMPTOMS

SUBJECTIVE: ■ Verbal complaints of difficulty in falling asleep ■ Verbal complaints of not feeling well rested ■ Awakening earlier or later than desired ■ Interrupted sleep ○ [Falls asleep during activities]

OBJECTIVE: ○ Changes in behavior and performance (increasing irritability, disorientation, listlessness, restlessness, lethargy) ○ Physical signs (mild, fleeting nystagmus, ptosis of eyelid, slight hand tremor, expressionless face, dark circles under eyes, changes in posture, frequent yawning) ○ Thick speech with mispronunciation and incorrect words

Social Interaction, impaired

DEFINITION: The state in which an individual participates in an insufficient or excessive quantity or ineffective quality of social exchange.   PROBLEM

RELATED FACTORS: ○ Knowledge/skill deficit about ways to enhance mutuality ○ Communication barriers [including head injury, stroke, other neurologic conditions affecting ability to communicate] ○ Self-concept disturbance ○ Absence of available significant other(s) or peers ○ Limited physical mobility [e.g., neuromuscular disease] ○ Therapeutic isolation ○ Sociocultural dissonance ○ Environmental barriers ○ Altered thought processes   ETIOLOGY

DEFINING CHARACTERISTICS   SIGNS
AND
SYMPTOMS

SUBJECTIVE: ■ Verbalized discomfort in social situations ■ Verbalized inability to receive or communicate a satisfying sense of belonging, caring, interest, or shared history ○ Family report of change of style or pattern of interaction

OBJECTIVE: ■ Observed discomfort in social situations ■ Observed inability to receive or communicate a satisfying sense of belonging, caring, interest,

---

■ = critical factors/major signs and symptoms
NOTE: Information appearing in [] has been added by the authors to clarify and facilitate the use of
nursing diagnoses.

or shared history ▪ Observed use of unsuccessful social interaction behaviors ▪ Dysfunctional interaction with peers, family, and/or others

Social Isolation

PROBLEM

DEFINITION: Aloneness experienced by the individual and perceived as imposed by others and as a negative or threatened state.

ETIOLOGY

RISK FACTORS: Factors contributing to the absence of satisfying personal relationships, such as: ○ Delay in accomplishing developmental tasks ○ Immature interests ○ Alterations in mental status ○ Altered state of wellness ○ Alterations in physical appearance ○ Unaccepted social behavior/values ○ Inadequate personal resources ○ Inability to engage in satisfying personal relationships ○ [Traumatic incidents or events]

SIGNS
AND
SYMPTOMS

DEFINING CHARACTERISTICS

SUBJECTIVE: ▪ Expresses feeling of aloneness imposed by others ▪ Expresses feelings of rejection ○ Expresses values acceptable to subculture but unacceptable to the dominant cultural group ○ Inability to meet expectations of others ○ Experiences feelings of difference from others ○ Inadequacy in or absence of significant purpose in life ○ Expresses interests inappropriate to development age/stage ○ Insecurity in public

OBJECTIVE: ▪ Absence of supportive significant other(s)—family, friends, group ○ Sad, dull affect ○ Inappropriate or immature interests/activities for developmental age/stage ○ Projects hostility in voice, behavior ○ Evidence of physical/mental handicap or altered state of wellness ○ Uncommunicative, withdrawn, no eye contact ○ Preoccupation with own thoughts, repetitive, meaningless actions ○ Seeks to be alone, or exists in subculture ○ Shows behavior unaccepted by dominant cultural group

Spiritual Distress (Distress of the Human Spirit)

PROBLEM

DEFINITION: Disruption in the life principle which pervades a person's entire being and which integrates and transcends one's biologic and psychosocial nature.

ETIOLOGY

RELATED FACTORS: ○ Separation from religious and cultural ties ○ Challenged belief and value system, for example, due to moral/ethical implications of therapy, due to intense suffering

SIGNS
AND
SYMPTOMS

DEFINING CHARACTERISTICS

SUBJECTIVE: ▪ Expresses concern with meaning of life/death and/or belief systems ○ Verbalizes inner conflict about beliefs; concern about relationship with deity; does not experience that God is forgiving ○ Questions moral/ethical implications of therapeutic regimen ○ Description of night-

---

▪ = critical factors/major signs and symptoms
NOTE: Information appearing in [] has been added by the authors to clarify and facilitate the use of nursing diagnoses.

mares/sleep disturbances ○ Anger toward God [as defined by the person]; displacement of anger toward religious representatives ○ Questions meaning of suffering ○ Questions meaning of own existence ○ Seeks spiritual assistance ○ Unable to choose [or chooses not] to participate in usual religious practices ○ [Regards illness as punishment] ○ [Unable to accept self; engages in self-blame] ○ [Description of somatic complaints]

OBJECTIVE: ○ Alteration in behavior or mood evidenced by anger, crying, withdrawal, preoccupation, anxiety, hostility, apathy, and so on ○ Gallows humor

Suffocation, high risk for*

DEFINITION: Accentuated risk of accidental suffocation (inadequate air available for inhalation).

PROBLEM

RISK FACTORS

ETIOLOGY

INTERNAL (INDIVIDUAL): ○ Reduced olfactory sensation ○ Reduced motor abilities ○ Lack of safety education; precautions ○ Cognitive or emotional difficulties [e.g., altered consciousness] ○ Disease or injury process

EXTERNAL (ENVIRONMENTAL): ○ Pillow/propped bottle placed in an infant's crib ○ Pacifier hung around infant's head ○ Children playing with plastic bags or inserting small objects into their mouths or noses ○ Children left unattended in bathtubs or pools ○ Discarded or unused refrigerators or freezers without removed doors ○ Vehicle warming in closed garage ○ Household gas leaks ○ Smoking in bed ○ Use of fuel-burning heaters not vented to outside ○ Low-strung clothesline ○ Eating of large mouthfuls of food

Swallowing, impaired

DEFINITION: The state in which an individual has decreased ability to voluntarily pass fluids and/or solids from the mouth to the stomach.

PROBLEM

RELATED FACTORS: ○ Neuromuscular impairment (e.g., decreased or absent gag reflex, decreased strength or excursion of muscles involved in mastication [and swallowing], perceptual impairment [decreased sensation in oral cavity], facial paralysis) ○ Mechanical obstruction (e.g., edema, tracheostomy tube, tumor) ○ Fatigue ○ Limited awareness ○ Reddened, irritated oropharyngeal cavity

ETIOLOGY

DEFINING CHARACTERISTICS

SIGNS AND SYMPTOMS

OBJECTIVE: ■ Observed evidence of difficulty in swallowing (e.g., stasis of food in oral cavity [pocketing/squirreling of food, food sticking], coughing/

■ = critical factors/major signs and symptoms
NOTE: Information appearing in [] has been added by the authors to clarify and facilitate the use of nursing diagnoses.
*[NOTE: A high risk diagnosis is *not* evidenced by signs and symptoms, since the problem has not yet occurred, and nursing interventions are directed at prevention. Therefore, risk factors which are present are noted instead.]

choking); [drooling, stranding phlegm, swallowing incoordination—repeated swallows, nasal regurgitation, wet/hoarse voice] ○ Evidence of aspiration, [foamy phlegm] ○ [Facial droop, difficulty chewing]

Thermoregulation, ineffective

PROBLEM

DEFINITION: The state in which the individual's temperature fluctuates between hypothermia and hyperthermia.

ETIOLOGY

RELATED FACTORS: ○ Trauma or illness [e.g., cerebral edema, cerebral vascular accident, intracranial surgery, or head injury] ○ Immaturity, aging [e.g., loss/absence of brown adipose tissue) ○ Fluctuating environmental temperature ○ [Changes in temperature of hypothalmic tissue causing alterations in emission of thermosensitive cells and regulation of heat loss/production] ○ [Changes in level/action of thyroxone and catecholamines] ○ [Changes in metabolic rate/activity] ○ [Chemical reactions in contracting muscles]

SIGNS
AND
SYMPTOMS

DEFINING CHARACTERISTICS:

OBJECTIVE: ■ Fluctuations in body temperature above or below the normal range.

Note: See also major and minor characteristics present in hypothermia and hyperthermia.

Thought Processes, altered

PROBLEM

DEFINITION: A state in which an individual experiences a disruption in cognitive operations and activities.

ETIOLOGY

RELATED FACTORS: ○ To be developed by NANDA ○ [Physiologic changes] ○ [Sleep deprivation] ○ [Psychologic conflicts]

SIGNS
AND
SYMPTOMS

DEFINING CHARACTERISTICS

SUBJECTIVE: ○ [Ideas of reference, hallucinations, delusions]

OBJECTIVE: ○ Inaccurate interpretation of environment ○ Memory deficit/problems, [disorientation to time, place, person, circumstances, and events] ○ Hyper/hypovigilance ○ Cognitive dissonance, [decreased ability to grasp ideas, make decisions, problem-solve; reason, abstract or conceptualize, calculate] ○ Distractibility, [altered attention span] ○ Egocentricity ○ [Confabulation] ○ [Inappropriate social behavior]

OTHER POSSIBLE CHARACTERISTICS: ○ Inappropriate/nonreality-based thinking

---

■ = critical factors/major signs and symptoms
NOTE: Information appearing in [] has been added by the authors to clarify and facilitate the use of nursing diagnoses.

Tissue Integrity, impaired

DEFINITION: A state in which an individual experiences damage to mucous membrane, or corneal, integumentary, or subcutaneous tissue.

PROBLEM

RELATED FACTORS: ○ Altered circulation ○ Nutritional deficit/excess ○ Fluid deficit/excess ○ Knowledge deficit ○ Impaired physical mobility ○ Irritants, chemical (including body excretions, secretions, medications) ○ Thermal (temperature extremes) ○ Mechanical (pressure, shear, friction), radiation (including therapeutic radiation)

ETIOLOGY

DEFINING CHARACTERISTICS

SIGNS AND SYMPTOMS

OBJECTIVE: ■ Damaged or destroyed tissue (cornea, mucous membrane, integumentary, or subcutaneous)

Tissue Perfusion, altered, (specify type) Cerebral, Cardiopulmonary, Renal, Gastrointestinal, Peripheral

DEFINITION: The state in which an individual experiences a decrease in nutrition and oxygenation at the cellular level due to a deficit in capillary blood supply. [Tissue perfusion problems can exist without decreased cardiac output; however, there may be a relationship between cardiac output and tissue perfusion.]

PROBLEM

ETIOLOGY: ○ Interruption of flow, arterial; venous ○ Exchange problems ○ Hypervolemia; hypovolemia

ETIOLOGY

DEFINING CHARACTERISTICS

SIGNS AND SYMPTOMS

SUBJECTIVE: ○ Claudication ○ [Angina] ○ [Palpitations]

OBJECTIVE: ■ Diminished/[absent] arterial pulsations ○ Skin color: ■ Pale on elevation, color does not return on lowering leg; ○ dependent, blue or purple, [or mottled] ○ Skin temperature, cold extremities ○ Skin quality: shining, lack of lanugo ○ Blood pressure changes in extremities ○ Bruits ○ Slow-growing, dry, thick brittle nails ○ Slow healing of lesions ○ Round scars covered with atrophied skin ○ Gangrene ○ [Delayed capillary refill]

(Further work and development are required for the subcomponents, specifically cerebral, renal, and gastrointestinal.)

CEREBRAL: ○ [Restlessness] ○ [Altered consciousness] ○ [Memory loss]

RENAL: ○ [Decreased urinary output] ○ [Edema formation] ○ [Hypertension]

GASTROINTESTINAL: ○ [Pain] ○ [Nausea/vomiting] ○ [Abdominal distention] ○ [Melena]

■ = critical factors/major signs and symptoms
NOTE: Information appearing in [] has been added by the authors to clarify and facilitate the use of nursing diagnoses.

Trauma, high risk for*

PROBLEM

DEFINITION: Accentuated risk of accidental tissue injury, for example, wound, burn, fracture.

ETIOLOGY

RISK FACTORS:

INTERNAL (INDIVIDUAL): ○ Weakness ○ Poor vision ○ Balancing difficulties ○ Reduced temperature and/or tactile sensation ○ Reduced large, or small, muscle coordination/hand–eye coordination ○ Lack of safety education/precautions ○ Insufficient finances to purchase safety equipment or effect repairs ○ Cognitive or emotional difficulties ○ History of previous trauma

EXTERNAL (ENVIRONMENTAL) [includes but is not limited to]: ○ Slippery floors, for example, wet or highly waxed ○ Snow or ice collected on stairs, walkways; unanchored rugs ○ Bathtub without hand grip or antislip equipment ○ Use of unsteady ladder or chairs ○ Entering unlighted rooms ○ Unsturdy or absent stair rails ○ Unanchored electric wires ○ Litter or liquid spills on floors or stairways ○ High beds ○ Children playing without gates at top of stairs ○ Obstructed passageways ○ Unsafe window protection in homes with young children ○ Inappropriate call-for-aid mechanisms for bed-resting client ○ Pot handles facing toward front of stove ○ Bathing in very hot water, for example, unsupervised bathing of young children ○ Potential igniting gas leaks ○ Delayed lighting of gas burner or oven ○ Experimenting with chemical or gasoline ○ Unscreened fires or heaters ○ Wearing plastic apron or flowing clothing around open flame ○ Children playing with matches, candles, cigarettes ○ Inadequately stored combustibles or corrosives, for example, matches, oily rags, lye ○ Highly flammable children's toys or clothing ○ Overloaded fuse boxes ○ Contact with rapidly moving machinery, industrial belts, or pulleys ○ Sliding on coarse bed linen or struggling within bed restraints ○ Faulty electric plugs, frayed wires, or defective appliances ○ Contact with acids or alkalis ○ Playing with fireworks or gunpowder ○ Contact with intense cold ○ Overexposure to sun, sun lamps, radiotherapy ○ Use of cracked dishware or glasses ○ Knives stored uncovered ○ Guns or ammunition stored unlocked ○ Large icicles hanging from roof ○ Exposure to dangerous machinery ○ Children playing with sharp-edged toys ○ High-crime neighborhood and vulnerable clients ○ Driving a mechanically unsafe vehicle ○ Driving after partaking of alcoholic beverages or drugs ○ Driving at excessive speeds ○ Driving without necessary visual aids ○ Children riding in the front seat of car ○ Smoking in bed or near oxygen ○ Overloaded electric outlets ○ Grease waste collected on stoves ○ Use of thin or worn pot holders [or mitts] ○ Nonuse or misuse of necessary headgear for motorized cyclists or young children carried on adult bicycles ○ Unsafe road or road-crossing conditions ○ Play or work near vehi-

---

■ = critical factors/major signs and symptoms
NOTE: Information appearing in [] has been added by the authors to clarify and facilitate the use of nursing diagnoses.
*[**NOTE:** A high risk diagnosis is *not* evidenced by signs and symptoms, since the problem has not yet occurred, and nursing interventions are directed at prevention. Therefore, risk factors which are present are noted instead.]

cle pathways, for example, driveways, lanes, railroad tracks ○ Nonuse or misuse of seat restraints/[unrestrained infants/children riding in car]

Unilateral Neglect

DEFINITION: A state in which an individual is perceptually unaware of and inattentive to one side of the body [and the immediate unilateral territory/space].

PROBLEM

RELATED FACTORS: ○ Effects of disturbed perceptual abilities, for example, [homonymous] hemianopsia; [or visual inattention] ○ One-sided blindness; neurologic illness or trauma ○ [Impaired cerebral blood flow]

ETIOLOGY

DEFINING CHARACTERISTICS

SIGNS AND SYMPTOMS

SUBJECTIVE: ○ [Complaints of feeling that part does not belong to own self]

OBJECTIVE: ■ Consistent inattention to stimuli on an affected side [■] Inadequate self-care [inability to satisfactorily perform activities of daily living] ○ Positioning and/or safety precautions in regard to the affected side ○ Does not look toward affected side ○ Leaves food on plate on the affected side ○ [Does not touch affected side] ○ [Failure to use the affected side of the body without being reminded to do so]

Urinary Elimination, altered

DEFINITION: The state in which an individual experiences a disturbance in urine elimination.

PROBLEM

RELATED FACTORS: Multiple causality, including: ○ Sensory motor impairment ○ Anatomical obstruction ○ Urinary tract infection ○ Mechanical trauma ○ [Surgical diversion]

ETIOLOGY

DEFINING CHARACTERISTICS

SIGNS AND SYMPTOMS

SUBJECTIVE: ○ Frequency ○ Hesitancy ○ Dysuria

OBJECTIVE: ○ Nocturia ○ Urgency ○ Incontinence ○ Retention

Urinary Retention [Acute/Chronic]

DEFINITION: The state in which the individual experiences incomplete emptying of the bladder. [High urethral pressure inhibits voiding until increased abdominal pressure causes urine to be involuntarily lost, or high urethral pressure inhibits complete emptying of bladder.]

PROBLEM

RELATED FACTORS: ○ High urethral pressure caused by weak detrusor [absent detrusor] ○ Inhibition of reflex arc ○ Strong sphinctor; blockage [e.g., BPH, perineal swelling] ○ [Habituation of reflex arc] ○ [Use of medications with

ETIOLOGY

■ = critical factors/major signs and symptoms

NOTE: Information appearing in [] has been added by the authors to clarify and facilitate the use of nursing diagnoses.

side-effect of retention, e.g., atropine, belladonna, psychotropics, antihistamines, opiates]

SIGNS
AND
SYMPTOMS

DEFINING CHARACTERISTICS

SUBJECTIVE: ○ Sensation of bladder fullness ○ Dribbling ○ Dysuria

OBJECTIVE: ■ Bladder distention ■ Small, frequent voiding or absence of urine output ○ Residual urine [150 ml or more] ○ Overflow incontinence ○ [Reduced stream]

Violence [Actual], high risk for: directed at Self/Others*

PROBLEM

DEFINITION: A state in which an individual experiences behaviors that can be physically harmful either to the self or others. [The "harm" can range from neglect to abuse or even death and may be psychologic and/or physical.]

ETIOLOGY

RELATED FACTORS [FOR "ACTUAL" DIAGNOSIS]: ○ Antisocial character ○ Catatonic/manic excitement ○ Panic states, rage reactions ○ Suicidal behavior ○ Toxic reactions to medication [including illicit drugs/alcohol] ○ Battered women [spouse abuse]; child abuse ○ Organic brain syndrome; temporal lobe epilepsy ○ [Negative role modeling] ○ [Developmental crisis] ○ [Hormone imbalance, e.g., PMS, postpartal depression/psychosis]

RISK FACTORS [OR DEFINING CHARACTERISTICS FOR "ACTUAL" DIAGNOSIS]: ○ Body language: (clenched fists, tense facial expressions, rigid posture, tautness indicating effort to control) ○ Overt and aggressive acts (goal-directed destruction of objects in environment) ○ Self-destructive behavior, active aggressive suicidal acts ○ Hostile threatening verbalizations (boasting to or prior abuse of others) ○ Increased motor activity (pacing, excitement, irritability, agitation) ○ Possession of destructive means (gun, knife, weapon) ○ Suspicion of others, paranoid ideation, delusions, hallucinations ○ Substance abuse/withdrawal ○ Rage ○ [Expresses intent/desire to harm self or others, directly or indirectly]

OTHER POSSIBLE CHARACTERISTICS:

Inability to verbalize feelings;
Provocative behavior: (argumentative, dissatisfied, overreactive, hypersensitive);
Fear of self or others;
Vulnerable self-esteem;
Anger;
Repetition of verbalizations (continued complaints, requests, and demands);
Increasing anxiety level; and/or
Depression (specifically active, aggressive, suicidal acts)

■ = critical factors/major signs and symptoms
NOTE: Information appearing in [] has been added by the authors to clarify and facilitate the use of nursing diagnoses.
*[**NOTE:** A high risk diagnosis is *not* evidenced by signs and symptoms, since the problem has not yet occurred, and nursing interventions are directed at prevention. Therefore, risk factors which are present are noted instead.]

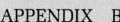

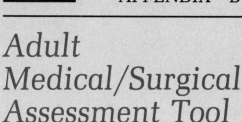

Adult Medical/Surgical Assessment Tool

This is a suggested guide/tool for development by an individual or institution to create a database reflecting Diagnostic Divisions of Nursing Diagnoses. Although the divisions are alphabetized for ease of presentation, they can be prioritized or rearranged to meet individual needs.

General Information

Name; Age; DOB; Sex; Race; Admission Date, Time, From; Source of Information, Reliability (1–4 with 4 = very reliable).

ACTIVITY/REST
Subjective

Occupation; usual activities/hobbies; leisure time activities.
Complaints of boredom; limitations imposed by condition.
Sleep: # of hours, naps, aids; insomnia, related to; rested upon awakening.

Objective

Observed response to activity: cardiovascular, respiratory.
Mental status (i.e., withdrawn/lethargic).
Neuro/muscular assessment: muscle mass/tone, posture, tremors, ROM, strength, deformity.

CIRCULATION
Subjective

History of: hypertension, heart trouble, rheumatic fever, ankle/leg edema, phlebitis, slow healing, claudication.
Extremities: numbness, tingling. Cough/hemoptysis.
Change in frequency/amount of urine.

Objective

B/P: R and L: lying/sit/stand, pulse pressure, ausculatory gap.

Pulse (palpation): carotid, temporal, jugular, radial, femoral, popliteal, post tibial, dorsalis pedis.

Cardiac (palpation): PMI, thrill, heaves. Heart sounds: rate, rhythm, quality, friction rub, murmur.

Breath sounds: vascular bruit. Jugular vein distention.

Extremities: temperature, color, capillary refill, Homan's sign, varicosities, nails (abnormalities), distribution/quality of hair. Color/cyanosis: overall, mucous membranes, lips, nail beds, conjunctiva, sclera, diaphoresis.

EGO INTEGRITY

Subjective

Report of stress factors; ways of handing stress; financial concerns; relationship status; cultural factors; religion, practicing; lifestyle, recent changes.

Feelings of: helplessness, hopelessness, powerlessness.

Objective

Emotional status: calm, anxious, angry, withdrawn, fearful, irritable, restive, euphoric. Observed physiologic response(s).

ELIMINATION

Subjective

Usual bowel pattern; laxative use; character of stool; last BM; history of bleeding; hemorrhoids; constipation; diarrhea.

Usual voiding pattern; incontinence/when, urgency, frequency, retention; character of urine; pain/burning/difficulty voiding; history of kidney/bladder disease; diuretic use.

Objective

Abdomen tender, soft/firm, palpable mass, size/girth, bowel sounds; hemorrhoids; bladder palpable; overflow voiding.

FOOD/FLUID

Subjective

Usual diet (type), # meals daily; last meal/intake; dietary pattern.

Loss of appetite; nausea/vomiting; heartburn/indigestion, related to, relieved by; allergy/food intolerance.

Mastication/swallowing problems, dentures.

Usual weight, changes in weight. Diuretic use.

Objective

Current weight; height; body build. Skin turgor; mucous membranes moist/dry. Hernia/masses. Edema: general, dependent, periorbital, ascites; jugular vein distention. Thyroid enlarged.

Halitosis; condition of teeth/gums; appearance of tongue, mucous membranes.

Bowel sounds; breath sounds; urine S/A or Chemstix.

HYGIENE
Subjective

Activities of daily living: independent/dependent—mobility, feeding, hygiene, dressing, toileting, other.

Equipment/prosthetic devices required; assistance provided by.

Preferred time of bath.

Objective

General appearance; manner of dress; personal habits; body odor; condition of scalp; presence of vermin.

NEUROSURGERY
Subjective

Fainting spells/dizziness; headaches: location, frequency; tingling/numbness/weakness (location). Stroke (residual effects).

Seizures, aura, how controlled.

Eyes: vision loss, last exam, glaucoma, cataract.

Ears: hearing loss, last exam.

Epistaxis; sense of smell.

Objective

Mental status: oriented/disoriented: time, place, person, alert, drowsy, lethargic, stuporous, comatose, cooperative, combative, delusions, hallucinations, affect (describe).

Memory: recent, remote.

Glasses, contacts; hearing aids.

Pupil size/reaction: R/L; facial droop; swallowing; handgrasp/release: R/L; posturing; deep tendon reflexes; paralysis.

PAIN/DISCOMFORT
Subjective

Location, intensity (1–10 with 10 most severe), frequency, quality, duration, radiation, precipitating factors, how relieved; associated symptoms.

Objective

Facial grimacing; guarding affected area; emotional response; narrowed focus.

RESPIRATION
Subjective

Dyspnea, related to; cough/sputum.

History of bronchitis, asthma, tuberculosis, emphysema, recurrent pneumonia, other, exposure to noxious fumes.

Smoker, pk/day, # of years; use of respiratory aids; oxygen.

Objective

Respiratory: rate, depth, symmetry, use of accessory muscles, nasal flaring; fremitis. Breath sounds; egophony. Cyanosis; clubbing of fingers. Sputum characteristics. Mentation/restlessness.

SAFETY
Subjective

Allergies/sensitivities, reaction; previous alteration of immune system, cause. History of sexually transmitted disease (date/type); high risk behaviors; testing; blood transfusion/number, when, reaction, described.

History of accidental injuries; fractures/dislocations; arthritis/unstable joints; back problems. Changes in moles; enlarged nodes. Impaired: vision, hearing. Prosthesis; ambulatory devices.

Objective

Temperature; diaphoresis.

Skin integrity, scars, rashes, lacerations, ulcerations, ecchymosis, blisters, burns, degree/percent. Drainage.

General strength, muscle tone, gait, ROM, paresthesia/paralysis.

Results of cultures, immune system testing.

SEXUALITY: [COMPONENT OF SOCIAL INTERACTION]

Sexually active; use of condoms; sexual concerns/difficulties; recent change in frequency/interest.

Female

Subjective

Age at menarche, length of cycle, duration, last menstrual period, menopause; vaginal discharge; bleeding between periods.

Practices breast self-exam; last PAP smear.

Objective

Breast exam; vaginal warts/lesions.

Male

Subjective

Penile discharge; prostate disorder; circumcised; vasectomy.

Practice self-exam: breast/testicles; last proctoscopic/prostate exam.

Objective

Exam: breast/penis/testicles.

SOCIAL INTERACTIONS

Subjective

Martial status, years in relationship, living with, concerns/stresses.

Extended family; other support person(s). Role within family structure. Report of problems related to illness/condition.

Change in speech, laryngectomy.

Objective

Speech: clear, slurred, unintelligible; aphasic; unusual speech pattern/impairment. Use of speech aids.

Verbal/nonverbal communication with family/significant other(s); family interaction (behavioral) pattern.

TEACHING/LEARNING

Subjective

Dominant language (specify); literate; education level; learning disabilities (specify); cognitive limitations.

Health beliefs/practices; special healthcare practices.

Familial risk factors (indicate relationship): diabetes, tuberculosis, heart disease, strokes, high B/P, epilepsy, kidney disease, cancer, mental illness, other.

Prescribed medications: drug, dose, times, take regularly, purpose; non-prescription drugs: over-the-counter (OTC), street drugs; smokeless tobacco; use of alcohol (amount/frequency).

Admitting diagnosis per physician; reason for hospitalization per patient; history of current complaint; patient expectations of this hospitalization; previous illnesses and/or hospitalizations/surgeries; evidence of failure to improve; last complete physical exam.

DISCHARGE PLAN CONSIDERATIONS

Date information obtained; anticipated date of discharge. Resources available: persons, financial. Anticipate changes in living situation after discharge; areas that may require alteration/assistance: food preparation, shopping, transportation, ambulation, medication/IV therapy, treatments, wound care, supplies, self-care assistance (specify); physical layout of home; homemaker assistance; living facility other than home (specify).

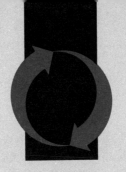

NANDA Nursing Diagnoses Organized According to Maslow's Hierarchy of Needs

SELF-ACTUALIZATION

Family Coping, potential for growth
Growth and Development, altered
Health Seeking Behaviors
Spiritual Distress

SELF-ESTEEM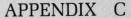

Adjustment, impaired
Body Image disturbance
Coping, defensive
Coping, ineffective individual
Decisional conflict
Denial, ineffective
Diversional Activity deficit
Hopelessness
Noncompliance
Nutrition, altered, more than body needs
Personal Identity disturbance
Post-trauma response
Powerlessness
Rape-Trauma syndrome
Self-esteem, chronic low
Self-esteem disturbance

Self-esteem, situational low
Violence, high risk

LOVE AND BELONGING

Family coping, ineffective, compromised/disabling
Family processes, altered
Parenting, altered
Parental role conflict
Role Performance, altered
Social Interaction impairment
Social Isolation

SAFETY AND SECURITY

Anxiety
Communication, impaired verbal
Disuse Syndrome, high risk
Dysreflexia
Fear
Grieving, anticipatory
Grieving, dysfunctional
Health Maintenance Management, impaired
Home Maintenance Management, impaired
Infection, high risk
Injury, high risk
Knowledge deficit
Poisoning, high risk
Protection, altered
Trauma, high risk
Unilateral Neglect

PHYSIOLOGIC NEEDS

Activity intolerance
Airway clearance, ineffective
Aspiration, high risk
Body temperature altered, high risk
Breastfeeding, effective
Breastfeeding, ineffective
Breathing Pattern, ineffective
Cardiac Output, decreased
Constipation, colonic/perceived
Diarrhea
Fatigue
Fluid Volume deficit
Fluid Volume excess
Gas Exchange impairment
Hyperthermia
Hypothermia
Incontinence, bowel/functional/reflex/stress/total/urge

Nutrition, altered, less than body requirements
Oral Mucous Membrane, altered
Pain
Pain, chronic
Physical Mobility, impairment
Protection, altered
Self-care deficit (specify)
Sensory-perceptual alteration
Sexual dysfunction
Sexuality Pattern, altered
Skin Integrity, impaired
Sleep Pattern disturbance
Suffocation, potential
Swallowing, impaired
Thermoregulation, ineffective
Thought Processes, altered
Tissue Integrity, impaired
Tissue Perfusion, altered
Urinary Elimination, altered patterns
Urinary retention

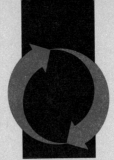

Diagnostic Qualifiers

Actual Nursing Diagnosis

(LABEL)

This part provides a name for the diagnosis, a concise phrase or term that represents a pattern of related cues.

High Risk Nursing Diagnosis (formerly potential)

(LABEL)

This part provides a name for the diagnosis, a concise phrase or term that represents a pattern of related cues.

Diagnostic labels may include but are not limited to the following qualifiers:

IMPAIRED

Made worse, weakened; damaged, reduced; deteriorated.

DEPLETED

Emptied wholly or partially; exhausted of.

DEFICIENT

Inadequate in amount, quality, or degree; defective; not sufficient; incomplete.

191

EXCESSIVE

Characterized by an amount or quantity that is greater than is necessary, desirable, or usable.

DYSFUNCTIONAL

Abnormal; impaired or incompletely functioning.

DISTURBED

Agitated; interrupted, interfered with.

ACUTE

Severe but of short duration.

CHRONIC

Lasting a long time; recurring; habitual; constant.

INTERMITTENT

Stopping and starting again at intervals; periodic; cyclic.

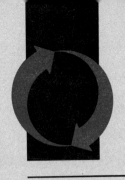

Common Medical, Charting, and Prescription Abbreviations†

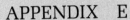

MEDICAL ABBREVIATIONS

ABBREVIATION	DEFINITION
ad	to; up to
ad lib.	freely; at pleasure
ALT	alanine aminotransferase (formerly SGPT)
AQ	water
AST	aspartate aminotransferase (formerly SGOT)
AV	atrioventricular
av	avoirdupois
B P	British Pharmacopeia
BUN	blood urea nitrogen
C	Calorie (kilocalorie); Celsius; centigrade
ca.	gallon
CBC	complete blood count
cc.	cubic centimeter
CDC	Centers for Disease Control
cg.	centigram
cm	centimeter
comp	compound
CNS.	central nervous system
cong	gallon
CSF	cerebrospinal fluid
CV	cardiovascular
d	right; day (24 hours)
/d	per day

ABBREVIATION	DEFINITION
D&C	dilatation and curettage
DPT	diphtheria-pertussis-tetanus
dr.	dram
ECG	electrocardiogram
ECT	electroconvulsive therapy
EEG	electroencephalogram
elix	elixir
EMG	electromyogram
emp	a plaster
ENT	ear, nose, and throat
ESR	erythrocyte sedimentation rate
F	Fahrenheit
f	female
FDA	Food and Drug Administration
FEV	forced expiratory volume
Fld	fluid
fl dr	fluidram
fl oz	fluidounce
FSH	follicle-stimulating hormone
GI	gastrointestinal
Gm; gm	gram
gr	grain

† Adapted from Thomas, CL (ed): Taber's Cyclopedic Medical Dictionary, ed 16. FA Davis, Philadelphia, 1989, with permission.

MEDICAL ABBREVIATIONS (*continued*)

ABBREVIATION	DEFINITION
Gtt; gtt	drops
h	hour
hgb	hemoglobin
IM	intramuscular
inf	infusion
inhal	inhalation
inj	injection
instill	instillation
IQ	intelligence quotient
IU	international unit
IUD	intrauterine device
IV	intravenously
kg	kilogram
l	liter
lab	laboratory
lb	pound
LD50	lethal dose, median
liq	liquid; fluid
m	male; meter; minim
MED	minimum effective dose
mEq	milliequivalent
mg	milligram
ml	milliliter
mM	millimole
mm	millimeter
mol wt	molecular weight
mph	miles per hour
MPN	most probable number
μEq	microequivalent
μg	microgram
no	number
NPN	nonprotein nitrogen
O	pint
OC	oral contraceptive
O D	right eye
O L	left eye
O S	left eye

ABBREVIATION	DEFINITION
oz	ounce
paren	parenterally
PBI	protein-bound iodine
pH	hydrogen ion concentration
ppm	parta per million
pt	pint
qt	quart
rad	radiation absorbed dose
s	without
S	mark
s c	subcutaneously
s cut	subcutaneously
SGOT	serum glutamic oxaloacetic transaminase (see AST)
SGPT	serum glutamic pyruvic transaminase (see ALT)
sp gr	specific gravity
spt	spirit
s q	subcutaneously
stat	immediately
syr	syrup
top	topically
tr, tinct	tincture
UHF	Ultra High Frequency
ung	ointment
UV	ultraviolet
vin	wine
Vo_2	maximum oxygen consumption
vol %	volume percent
WBC	white blood count
Wt	weight
w/v	weight in volume
x	multiplied by

CHARTING ABBREVIATIONS

ABBREVIATION	DEFINITION
abs feb	without fever
a c	before a meal
ad effect	to effect
adhib	to be administered
ad lib	at pleasure
ad part dolent	to the aching part
adst feb	when fever is present
ad us	according to custom
ad us ext	for external use
af feb	when the fever increases
alt dieb	every other day

ABBREVIATION	DEFINITION
alt hor	every other hour
alt noc	every other night
aq	water
bal	bath
bal sin	mustard bath
bis in 7d	twice a week
BP	blood pressure
$\bar{c}$	with
cat	a poultice
cito disp	let it be dispensed quickly

CHARTING ABBREVIATIONS (*continued*)

ABBREVIATION	DEFINITION
c m	tomorrow morning
c m s	to be taken tomorrow morning
cont rem	let the medicine be continued
c v	tomorrow evening
cyath	ladle (wineglass)
cyath vinos	wineglass
d	give
d	day
/d	per day
decub	lying down
donec alv sol ft	until the bowels are open
dur dolor	while pain lasts
en, enem	enema
exhib	let it be displayed
h n	tonight
hor som, h s	bedtime
in d	daily
mod praesc	as prescribed
mor dict	in the manner directed
mor sol	in the usual manner
n b	note well
noct	of the night
n p o	nothing by mouth
p	after

ABBREVIATION	DEFINITION
p a a	let it be applied to the affected region
post cib or p c	after meals
p r	through the rectum
p r n	as needed
Q h	every hour
Q 2h	every two hours
Q 3h	every three hours
q i d	four times a day
q l	as much as wanted
q p	as much as desired
q s	as much as may be needed
quotid	quotidie
s	without
s a or sec a	by skill
semih	half an hour
s o s	if necessary
st	let it (them) stand
sum	let him take; to be taken
s v	alcoholic spirit
s v v	brandy
T	temperature
ter	rub
t i d	three times a day
t i n	three times a night
ur	urine

PRESCRIPTION ABBREVIATIONS

ABBREVIATION	DEFINITION
a̅a̅ or a	of each
add	add
adhib	to be administered
admov	supply
ad sat	to saturation
aeq	equals
agit	shake; stir
agit ante sum	shake before taking
alb	white
aq bull	boiling water
aq cal	hot water
aq dest	distilled water
aq ferv	boiling water
aq font	spring water
aq frig	cold water
aq menth pip	peppermint water
aq pur	pure water
bib	drink
b i d	twice daily
b i n	twice a night
bol	a pill
bull	let it boil

ABBREVIATION	DEFINITION
c̅	with
cap	a capsule
chart or cht	a small medicated paper
coch mag	a large spoonful
coch med	a half spoonful
coch parv	a teaspoonful
collyr	an eyewash
comp	compound of
cuj lib	of any you please
D	dose
d	give
d d in d	from day to day
dec	pour off
dent tal dos	give of such doses
det	let it be given
dieb alt	every other day
dieb tert	every 3rd day
dil	dilute, diluted
dim	halved
div	divide
div in p aeq	let it be halved into equal parts

PRESCRIPTION ABBREVIATIONS (*continued*)

ABBREVIATION	DEFINITION
donec alv sol ft	until the bowels are open
dos	dose
dur dolor	while pain lasts
e m p	as directed
emp	a plaster
emuls	an emulsion
epistom	a stopper
ect	to speed; extract
ferv	boiling
f h	let a draught be made
filt	filter
f m	let a mixture be made
f p	let a potion be made
f pil	let a pill be made
ft	let it be made
garg	a gargle
grad	by degrees
gtt	drops
guttat	drop by drop
haust	a draught
hor decub	at bedtime
hor som or h s	at bedtime
hor 1 spat	one hour's time
inf	an infusion
int	to be innermost
lin	a liniment
liq	a solution
lot	a lotion
M.	mix
mac	soften
man prim	first thing in the morning
mas	a mass
med	a medicine
m et n	morning and night
mist	a misture
mitt	let go
mitt x tal	send ten like this
mod	moderate-sized
mod praesc	in the manner prescribed
moll	soft
mor dict	in the manner directed
mor sol	as accustomed

ABBREVIATION	DEFINITION
ne tr s num	deliver not without the money
no	number
noct maneq	night and morning
non rep, n r	do not repeat
omn bid	every 2 days
omn bih	every 2 hours
omn hor	every hour
omn noct	every night
om 1/4 h	every 15 minutes
om mane vel noc	every morning or night
part aeq	equal parts
part vic	in divided doses
p c	after meals
pil	a pill
p o	by mouth
p p a	the bottle having first been shaken
pro rat aet	according to patient's age
pulv	powder
red in pulv	reduced to powder
repetat, rep	let it be repeated
rub	red
sig	write; let it be labeled
sing	of each
sol	a solution
solv	dissolve
ss	a half
subind	immediately after
sum	take
sum tal	take 1 like this
suppos	a suppository
s v r	rectified spirit of wine
tab	a medicated tablet
tinct	a tincture
trit	triturate or grind
ult praes	the last ordered
ung	ointment
ut dict	as directed
vitel	yolk of an egg

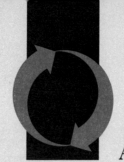

Key to Practice Activities and Work Pages

KEY TO PRACTICE ACTIVITY 2-1

1. Skin cool/damp: O; Sputum pale yellow: S or O; Allergic to eggs and sulfa: S; Pitting edema of feet and ankles: O; Usually voids 3 times per day: S; Chest pain lasting 15 minutes: S.
2. Column B: B, C, D, A, E.
3. Rewrite the following as open-ended questions:
   a. You're sad about what happened and are concerned about what you can do?
   b. I notice you seem to be in pain; tell me about it.
   c. I'd like to hear more about your interests, what you would enjoy doing.
   d. What is your understanding of what the doctor told you?
   e. Tell me about what you had for lunch.

KEY TO PRACTICE ACTIVITY 2-2

Diagnostic Divisions

Activity/Rest: 3, 11

Circulation: 8

Ego Integrity: 2, 10, 13

Elimination: 7

Food/Fluid: 6

Hygiene: 5

Neurosensory: 9

Pain/Comfort: 15

Respiration: 14

Safety: 4, 15

Sexuality: 1, 2

Social Interactions: 2

Teaching/Learning: 12

Functional Health Patterns

Health Perception/Health Management: 4, 12, 15

Nutritional/Metabolic: 6, 8, 14

Elimination: 7

Activity/Exercise: 4, 5

Cognitive/Perceptual: 9

Sleep/Rest: 11

Self-perception/Self-concept: 13

Role/Relationship: 1, 2, 3

Sexuality/Reproductive: 2

Coping/Stress Tolerance: 13

Value/Belief: 10

197

KEY TO PRACTICE ACTIVITY 3–1

Label P E S components (Questions 1 through 5).

1. P = Anxiety, severe
   E = changes in health status of fetus/self and threat of death
   S = restlessness, tremors, focus on self/fetus
2. P = Thought Processes, altered
   E = pharmacologic stimulation of the nervous system
   S = altered attention span, disorientation, and hallucinations
3. P = Coping, ineffective, individual
   E = maturational crisis
   S = inability to meet role expectations and alcohol abuse
4. P = Hyperthermia
   E = increased metabolic rate and dehydration
   S = elevated temperature, flushed skin, tachycardia, and tachypnea
5. P = Pain [acute]
   E = tissue distention and edema
   S = verbal complaints, guarding behavior, and changes in vital signs
6. An active diagnosis is one that is currently present and manifested by signs and symptoms. In recording the problem/need, you would use a three-part problem statement. A high risk diagnosis is one that you believe could develop, but since it has not occurred yet, there are no signs or symptoms, only "risk factors." Therefore the problem would be written as a two-part problem statement.
7. Active: Skin Integrity, impaired
   Pain [acute]
   Self-care deficit
   Knowledge deficit: treatment needs
   High risk: Infection, high risk for
   Adjustment impaired, high risk for
   Body image disturbance, high risk for

KEY TO PRACTICE ACTIVITY 3–2

1. Correct.
2. Correct.
3. Incorrect—related to medical diagnosis. In considering the pathophysiology of bronchitis, the underlying problem may actually be Airway Clearance, ineffective, related to excessive, thickened mucous secretions evidenced by rhonchi, dyspnea, and cyanosis.
4. Incorrect—related to and evidenced by statements are reversed.
5. Correct.

KEY TO PRACTICE ACTIVITY 4–1

a. 2, 4, 1, 3.
b. 1, 4, 2, 3.
c. 1, 4, 2, 3.

KEY TO PRACTICE ACTIVITY 4-2

Identify which of the following outcome statements are correctly written and modify those that are not.

1. Patient will: list individual risk factors and appropriate interventions.
   Incorrect—RATIONALE: There is no timeframe indicated.
   Corrected example: Patient will list individual risk factors and appropriate interventions within 72 hours.
2. Patient will: identify adaptive/protective measures for individual situation by discharge.
   Correct—RATIONALE: All elements of a measurable outcome are present.
3. Patient will: understand behaviors, lifestyle changes necessary to promote physical safety within 72 hours.
   Incorrect—RATIONALE: "Understands" is not a measurable verb.
   Corrected example: Patient will: verbalize understanding of behaviors, lifestyle changes necessary to promote physical safety within 72 hours.
4. Airway is patent, aspiration is prevented, ongoing.
   Incorrect—RATIONALE: There is no active verb; there is no subject.
   Corrected example: Patient will: maintain patent airway, ongoing.
   or
   Patient will: demonstrate techniques to prevent aspiration within 24 hours.
5. Patient will: assume responsibility for own learning by using available resources and participating in group discussion within 3 days.
   Correct—RATIONALE: All elements of a measurable outcome are present.

KEY TO PRACTICE ACTIVITY 4-3

Identify which interventions are correctly stated and rewrite those that are not.

1. Walk length of hall 2x/day with assistance. Correct
2. Force fluids.
   Incorrect—RATIONALE: The quantity of fluid is not indicated.
   Corrected example: Force fluid to a minimum of 2000 ml/day.
3. Pericare after each BM.
   Incorrect—RATIONALE: No verb and no indication of who is responsible for the activity.
   Corrected example: Provide [nurse], OR Assist with [nurse and patient] OR Encourage [patient] pericare after each bowel movement.
4. Encourage deep breathing exercises and cough q 2 h. Correct
5. Reduce environmental stimuli.
   Incorrect—RATIONALE: How/what?
   Corrected example: Maintain low lighting in room, OR Keep hallway door closed. . . .
6. Provide written handout for side-effects of medications prior to discharge.
   Correct

KEY TO PRACTICE ACTIVITY 4–4

Patient: Mike   Age 20   03/2/70   Sex M   Admitted 03/11/90   5:30 PM   Dx Compound Fx RTibia/Fibula

DATE	PATIENT DIAGNOSTIC STATEMENT	GOAL	INTERVENTIONS	OUTCOMES	STATUS
3/11/90	Pain, acute related to movement of bone fragments, soft tissue injury/edema evidenced by verbal complaints, guarding and muscle tension.	Free of pain by discharge.	1. Maintain limb rest R leg X24 h to 5 PM 3/12. 2. Elevate lower leg with folded blanket. 3. Apply ice to area as tol. X48 h to 5 PM 3/13. 4. Place cradle over foot of bed. 5. Document complaints and characteristics of pain. 6. Medicate with Demerol 75 mg & Vistaril 25mg—IM q4 h, PRN. 7. Demonstrate/encourage use of progressive relaxation techniques, deep breathing exercises, visualization. 8. Provide alternate comfort measures, position change, backrub. 9. Encourage use of diversional activities.	Verbalizes relief of pain within 30 min. of administration of meds. Identifies methods that provide relief by 3/12 9 AM. Uses relaxation skills to reduce level of pain by 3/12 9 AM.	

Signed: *Susan Hunter, RN*

KEY TO PRACTICE ACTIVITY 5-1

1. Organize interventions/activities:

Pt.	7	8	9	10	11	12	1	2	3	Comments
Martha	7:30-wt	VS Chair	Med	Shower Dressing		VS Chair	Med	I&O		

2. The plan will need to be reordered because Martha will need to be cleaned as quickly as possible.

For example: You may choose to give her a bath at this time depending on the extent of the problem. She may need to rest before she eats, and then you could give Martha her medications and rewarm her breakfast tray.

KEY TO PRACTICE ACTIVITY 5-2

1. a. written record
b. verbal report
2. Aids in verifying the status of invasive treatments, appearance of wounds/dressings, and the current condition of the patient.
3. Martha Ate well   Age 80   Dr. Jefferson
Weak and unsteady while up in hall   Dressing dry and intact
3 days postcholecystectomy   Scheduled for discharge tomorrow
Received oral pain medication at 11 AM with reported relief
Does not want to go home   Requires instruction in use of walker
Coordination for home care services in progress with the Discharge Planner
4. attending/primary physician; nursing supervisor; other nurses on your unit.

KEY TO PRACTICE ACTIVITY 6-1

Pain, acute   #2 M 3/12
#3 M 3/12

Although Mike is reporting relief of pain following administration of medication, this is an ongoing outcome and will remain active. Mike has identified methods that enhance pain relief and is successfully using relaxation techniques; thus the second and third outcomes have been met.

Infection, potential for   #1 M 3/12

Mike is able to identify and is practicing interventions to reduce risk of infection meeting the first outcome.

Physical Mobility   #1 M 3/12
#2 NM 3/12

Mike is participating in activities to maintain muscle strength meeting the first outcome. However, the initial attempt to get Mike out of bed was unsuccessful, and the second outcome is not met.

KEY TO PRACTICE ACTIVITY 6–2

Mike has learned ways to control his pain, and he seeks pharmacologic relief appropriately. The problem will remain active for the duration of this admission, although at a lesser level of concern. Intervention 1 can be deleted.

At this time, Mike's wounds show no signs of infection, and Mike is aware of ways to help reduce the risk of infection. Components of this problem will remain active for the duration of this hospitalization. Intervention 6 can be deleted.

Mike is able to reposition himself and participates in activities/behaviors to maintain function. Mike's initial attempt to be out of bed was not successful. The timeframe will need to be extended while Mike is evaluated for adequacy of circulation and appropriateness of premedication before activity is initiated again.

A problem of nutrition has also been identified. Verifying the integrity of Mike's jaws and teeth and providing a semisoft diet may help improve his intake. In addition, Mike's knowledge of his nutritional needs should be assessed, as a proper diet can promote healing and reduce risk of infection. A base-line weight should be obtained for future comparison.

KEY TO PRACTICE ACTIVITY 7–1

1. Recorded information can be reviewed by other staff members/health-care providers at any time.
2. Verifies implementation of the plan of treatment, events, activities, and progress toward outcomes.
3. Tracks the patient's responses to treatment, progress toward outcomes, and interventions used to obtain these outcomes to determine quality of care provided.
4. Meets standards necessary to gain accreditation.
5. A model for coworkers; gives an impression of abilities and identifies areas for additional training or supervision.
6. Proof of services necessary for payment.
7. Documents patient's interactions with others which may impact well-being, recovery, and independence.

KEY TO PRACTICE ACTIVITY 7–2

1. Mrs. Jewel has a poor body image since undergoing surgery. (J) For example: Mrs. Jewel says she thinks her husband will not want to look at her body, and she doesn't feel like a woman anymore.
2. Mr. Dunn needs to be evaluated regarding his competence to manage his household accounts because he is routinely receiving narcotic sedation. (O/B)
3. Miss Janus usually does her breast examination. (J) For example: Miss Janus does her breast examination monthly.
4. Mary Bird does not eat enough for her current level of activity. (J) For example: Mary Bird's caloric intake is only 1000 calories which represents maintenance level and is not sufficient to maintain her weight at her current level of activity.

5. Mrs. Lambert stops taking her medication; then when she has a seizure, she comes into the doctor's office for treatment. (O/B)

6. It has been a long time since Mr. Babbit has had his medications evaluated. (J) For example: Mr. Babbit has not had his medications evaluated since last November.

KEY TO WORK PAGE: CHAPTER ONE

1. The American Nurses Association has defined nursing as: The diagnosis and treatment of human responses to actual and potential health problems.

2. My own definition of nursing is: _____

   _____

3. The *ANA Social Policy Statement* defines the phenomena of concern for nurses as: human responses.

4. The definition of nursing process is: a five-step process providing an orderly, logical problem-solving approach for administering nursing care.

5. List and describe the five steps of the Nursing Process:
   a. Assessment: Systematic collection of data.
   b. Problem Identification: Analysis of data to identify patient's problems/needs.
   c. Planning: Setting goals/outcomes and choosing interventions.
   d. Implementation: Putting the plan into action.
   e. Evaluation: Assessing the effectiveness of the plan and changing the plan if indicated.

6. Choose three advantages of using the nursing process that you think are the most important:
   a. Provides framework for meeting individual needs of the patient, family, and community.
   b. Focuses attention on individual human responses to provide holistic care.
   c. Provides an organized, systematic method of problem-solving.
   d. Promotes active involvement of the patient.
   e. Enables the nurse to exert greater control over own practice.
   f. Provides a common language for practice.
   g. Provides a means for assessing nursing's economic contribution to patient care.

7. Identify three of the fundamental philosophical assumptions basic to decision-making within the nursing process:

   Patient is a human being who has worth and dignity.
   If basic human needs are not met, intervention is required until individual can resume responsibility for self.
   Patients have a right to quality health and nursing care with a focus on wellness and prevention.
   Therapeutic nurse-patient relationship is important to this process.

8. Identify the steps of the nursing process by numbering the appropriate

activity: 1—Assessment; 2—Problem identification; 3—Planning; 4—Implementation; and 5—Evaluation.

Robert, a 72-year-old male, is admitted with pneumonia. 1

He reports this is his second episode in 6 months. 1

Temperature is 101°F; skin hot and flushed. 1

He complains of frequent, hacking cough with moderate amount of thick greenish mucus. 1

Auscultation of the chest reveals scattered rhonchi throughout. 1

His mucous membranes are pale, and his lips are dry and cracked. 1

You determine that Robert has an ineffective airway clearance, a fluid volume deficit, and a knowledge deficit that will require teaching to promote adequate self-care and to prevent recurrence. 2

You establish the following outcomes:

Expectorates secretions completely with breath sounds clear and respirations noiseless. 3

Demonstrates adequate fluid balance with moist mucous membranes and loose respiratory secretions. 3

Verbalizes understanding of cause of condition and therapeutic regimen. 3

You decide to set up a regular schedule for respiratory activities and fluid replacement. 3

In addition, you formulate a teaching plan to cover the identified concerns for self-care and illness prevention. 3

You provide a tube of petroleum jelly for Robert to use on his lips. 4

Every 2 hours you visit Robert to encourage him to deep-breath, cough, change his position, and drink a glass of fluid of his choice. 4

You use this time to discuss avoidance of crowds and individuals with upper respiratory infections and recommend continuing the treatment plan after discharge. 4

The following day, Robert S.'s skin is no longer hot and flushed, temperature is 99°F, secretions are loose and readily expectorated, and breath sounds are clearing. 5

Robert S.'s lips and oral mucous membranes are moist. 5

He is able to explain in his own words how to care for himself and ways to prevent pneumonia. 5

You decide the current treatment plan is achieving the identified outcomes and to continue the plan as written. 5

KEY TO WORK PAGE: CHAPTER TWO

1. a. How was the respiratory treatment today?
   b. Tell me about your medication schedule. How is that working for you?
   c. Explain your understanding of these directions.
2. a. What do you think you need to do?
   b. I'm interested in what your concerns are.

   c. It seems difficult without him.

   d. I'd be interested in your thoughts about that.

3. In an emergency.

4. Nursing history, physical examination, and diagnostic studies.

5. Inspection; Percussion; Auscultation; Palpation.

6. The patient database is important to providing patient care because it provides a profile of the patient's health status on which problem identification is based.

7. Subjective data are what the patient/significant other(s) say that reflects their thoughts, feelings, perceptions. Objective data are observable and measurable and include data gathered from other sources.

8. Sally comes to the Obstetric Department for evaluation of her stage of labor. Back pains began about 3 hours ago during work as a respiratory therapist. Contractions are 5 minutes apart, lasting 40 seconds for the last 45 minutes. B/P 146/84, left arm/lying, pulse 110, respirations 24.

   Nauseated since a dinner of fried chicken 4 hours ago. Appears anxious and seems irritated that her physician is not here. Voided 1 hour ago, has not had a bowel movement for 2 days. Stopped smoking 8 months ago. Lungs clear. No allergies.

   Married, husband plans to attend the birth. Two children are in the care of their grandmother tonight. Appearance is well-groomed with a well fitting maternity uniform and low heeled shoes. Requests to leave contacts in to observe the birth. Last physical examination 1 week ago. Membranes have not ruptured. Due date is the middle of next week (2/25/90).

9. The benefit of doing "research" before an interview is to gather information and generate questions.

10. An interview should be "requested" because it promotes a more positive interaction.

11. Family/significant other; physician notes; old medical records; diagnostic studies; textbooks/reference journals; other nurses/healthcare providers.

12. Sensitivity of the nurse is important during the interview process to respect the patient's right to privacy and enhance trust.

13. Knowledge base; choice of questions to be asked; method of asking questions; ability to give meaning to responses; ability to synthesize the data; ability to prioritize the data.

14. Jennifer is a 3-year-old (1) female admitted to the outpatient surgery at 7 AM for (2) bilateral placement of tubes for chronic otitis media. (3) Has had nothing by mouth since midnight. (4) Uses diapers at night. (5) Voided at 6:30 AM—clear yellow. She says, (6) "My ear hurts," as she pulls on her right ear. (7) Thick, grayish yellow drainage present in the right ear. (8) Appears scared, clutching mother tightly and trembling. (9) Rectal temperature 98°F (36.5°C), (10) BP 85/48 (left arm/sitting), pulse 86/regular, (11) respirations 22/regular. (12) Skin warm, dry, color pink. (13) Right tympanic membrane dull, gray; perforation noted in central area. Mother reports, (14) "This is the second episode in two months." (15) Receiving Amoxicillin for the past week without improvement noted. In reviewing diagnostic studies, you note the (16) chest x-ray is clear, and a (17) culture of the drainage reveals streptococcus pneumoniae.

Diagnostic Divisions

Activity/Rest: none   Hygiene: 4   Safety: 7, 9, 17
Circulation: 10, 12   Neurosensory: 13   Sexuality: 1
Ego Integrity: 8   Pain/Comfort: 6   Social Interaction: none
Elimination: 5   Respiration: 11, 16 Teaching/Learning: 2,
Food/Fluid: 3   14, 15

KEY TO WORK PAGE: CHAPTER THREE

1. The process of data analysis using diagnostic reasoning to determine if nursing intervention is indicated.
2. The ANA Social Policy Statement and the ANA Standards of Practice.
3. a. Provides a common language for improved communication.
   b. Promotes identification of appropriate goals and interventions and provides guidance for evaluation.
   c. Provides framework for patient classification system for staffing needs and third-party reimbursement.
   d. Can be a standard for nursing practice.
   e. Provides opportunity for documentation and validation of process.

4. a. Problem-sensing
   b. Rule-out process
   c. Synthesizing data
   d. Evaluating/confirming the hypothesis
   e. List patient's problems/needs
   f. Reevaluate the problem list

5. a. Problem
   b. Etiology
   c. Signs/symptoms

6. Etiology and signs/symptoms are replaced by risk factors.
7. Medical diagnoses are illnesses/conditions while nursing diagnoses are human responses to actual and potential illnesses/conditions.
8. C/A: Knowledge deficit, drug therapy related to misinterpretation and unfamiliarity with resources as evidenced by request for information and statement of misconception.
   C/HR: High risk for Infection, related to altered lung expansion, decreased ciliary action, decreased hemoglobin, and invasive procedures.
   I/A: Urinary elimination, altered related to indwelling catheter evidenced by inability to void.
   C/A: Anxiety, moderate related to change in health status, role functioning, and socioeconomic status evidenced by apprehension, insomnia, and feelings of inadequacy.

9. Sally is visited by the Public Health Nurse for follow-up 6 days postdelivery. She complains about her bowels but says she has been drinking plenty of fluids, including fruit juices, and has been eating a balanced diet. Elimination section from the Patient Database

Subjective

Usual bowel patterns: every morning   **Laxative use:** rare/MOM pm

Character of stool: brown, formed   **Last BM:** <u>3 days ago</u>
   History of bleeding: No   **Hemorrhoids:** <u>last 5 weeks</u>
   Constipation: <u>since delivery</u>   **Diarrhea:** No
Usual voiding pattern: 3–4 x/day   **Incontinence:** No   **Urgency:** No
Character of urine: Yellow   **Pain/burning/difficulty voiding:** No
History of kidney/bladder disease: several bladder infections, <u>last one 6 years ago</u>
Associated complaints: <u>pain with stool, nausea, "I just can't go no matter what I do."</u>

Objective

Abdomen tender: <u>Yes</u>   **Soft/Firm:** <u>somewhat firm</u>
Palpable mass: No
   Size/girth: enlarged/postpartal
   Bowel sounds: present all 4 quadrants but <u>decreased</u>
Hemorrhoids: visual examination not done

Now write the Patient Diagnostic Statement: <u>Constipation related to weak abdominal musculature and pain on defecation evidenced by decreased frequency of stool, abdominal fullness, nausea, and decreased bowel sounds.</u>

KEY TO WORK PAGE: CHAPTER FOUR

1. <u>Provides continuity of care</u>
   <u>Enhances communication</u>
   <u>Assists with determining unit priorities</u>
   <u>Supports documentation of the nursing process</u>
   <u>Serves as a teaching tool</u>

2. Setting priorities is important <u>to assure that basic needs are met first, then other needs in order of importance.</u>

3. <u>A goal is stated broadly, reflecting the general direction in which the patient is expected to progress. An outcome is the measurable step taken toward achieving the goal.</u>

4. <u>(a) specific; (b) realistic; (c) consider the patient's circumstances and desires; (d) indicate a timeframe; (e) provide measurable evaluation criteria.</u>

5. <u>(a) date intervention is written; (b) action verb reflecting activity to be performed; (c) qualifiers of how, when, where, time/frequency, and amount; (d) signature and/or initials of the nurse.</u>

6. <u>Measurable verbs describe an action to be taken which can be observed and/or quantified, for example, "verbalizes," "ambulates"; and nonmeasurable verbs cannot be observed, for example, "understands."</u>

7. Discharge planning begins <u>when the patient is admitted.</u>

8. <u>The plan of care is documented on a single- or multipage form that is kept in a Kardex, in the patient's chart, or at the bedside.</u>

9. Identify two additional problems facing Mike, set a goal with one outcome and two interventions for each problem:

    a. Patient Diagnostic Statement: Infection, high risk for, related to broken skin, traumatized tissues, and insertion of pins.
        Goal: Free of infection.
        Outcome: Patient will: achieve timely wound healing free of purulent drainage and be afebrile—by discharge.
                                      or
        Outcome: Patient will: identify behaviors to reduce risk of infection within 24 hours.
        Interventions:

        - Monitor temperature/vital signs
        - Maintain aseptic technique with dressing change
        - Assess/document wound condition and pin sites
        - Administer antibiotic—monitor response
        - Instruct patient in ways to reduce risk of infection

    b. Patient Diagnostic Statement: Physical mobility, impaired, related to musculoskeletal impairment and pain as evidenced by reluctance to attempt movement and limited range of motion.
        Goal: Ambulates safely with assistive device.
        Outcome: Patient will: demonstrate techniques/behaviors that enable resumption of activities within 24 hours.
                                      or
        Outcome: Patient will: maintain position of function of the right leg/foot, free of foot drop—ongoing.
        Interventions:

        - Monitor circulation/nerve function of R leg
        - Position for optimum comfort as identified by patient
        - Support R leg with movement
        - Support foot in upright position with bed board/blanket roll

    c. Patient Diagnostic Statement: Knowledge deficit, self-care/treatment needs related to lack of previous exposure to information evidenced by request for information.
        Goal: Managing own care effectively.
        Outcome: Patient will: verbalize understanding of condition and treatment needs within 3 days.
        Outcome: Patient will: list signs/symptoms requiring medical evaluation/intervention, within 36 hours.
                                      or
        Outcome: Patient will: correctly perform wound/pin care and explain reasons for the actions.
        Interventions:

        - Review appropriate pathophysiology of injury in lay terms
        - Demonstrate proper wound and pin care
        - Identify signs/symptoms suggestive of complications
        - Discuss actions, side-effects, and possible adverse reactions to medications.

KEY TO WORK PAGE: CHAPTER FIVE

1. Identifying priorities, providing patient care, ongoing data collection, documentation, communication.
2. It is important to understand the expected effect and potential hazards of the interventions you will implement in order to be sure the intervention will be beneficial, that you are achieving the desired effects, or that you have allowed for changes necessary to provide for specific needs/safety.
3. Appropriateness of your action
   Need to alter interventions
   Development of new patient problems/needs
   Need for referral to other resources
   Necessity of shifting priorities to meet changing plans of care
4. a. Legal requirement for all healthcare settings
   b. Communication tool
5. "Hands-on" care; assisting the patient with care; instructing; counseling; monitoring.
6. The advantage of reporting "by exception" is that it provides for giving important information in a brief, concise manner to save time.
7. Patient confidentiality is important when discussing the patient in any area/situation where the conversation can be overheard by others who are not involved in the patient's care.

KEY TO WORK PAGE: CHAPTER SIX

1. Assessment identifies the patient's current status, and evaluation determines the patient's movement toward specified outcomes.
2. The primary purpose of the evaluation process is to determine how the plan of care is working.
3. a. Provides positive feedback to patient and nurse
   b. Provides encouragement to continue to strive for higher level of functioning
   c. Provides for problem-solving and personal growth
4. a. Direct observation. Ambulated the length of the hall.
   b. Patient interview. Reports decreased level of pain.
   c. Review of records. Temperature has remained within normal range.
5. Since it is advisable to deal with only three to five nursing diagnoses, needs are prioritized according to the hierarchy of needs, meeting basic needs first.
6. Consideration of discharge planning is begun on admission.
7. a. **Evaluation:** Based on the above information, evaluate Donald's progress regarding his problems of Nutrition, less than body requirements, Coping, ineffective, and Role Performance, altered.

   Problem 4: Donald's intake is meeting daily caloric requirements, achieving the second outcome. However, his menu choices do not include all food groups appropriately; therefore the first outcome is only partially met.

   Problem 5: Donald recognizes the impact that his loss of employment and recent divorce have had on his current feelings of anxiety and helplessness, meeting the first outcome.

Problem 6: Donald is expressing awareness of feelings related to his situation and has some optimism for the future. This meets the first outcome. In addition, Donald has developed a realistic plan with two job-hunting strategies, meeting the second outcome.

b. **Modification:** How would you change Donald's plan of care? Investigate Donald's menu choices and how he plans to meet dietary needs without adequate intake of fruits and vegetables.

c. How might new concerns regarding the patient affect your discharge plans? Identify a contact person from AA to provide support for Donald to promote continued involvement in the treatment plan.

KEY TO WORK PAGE: CHAPTER SEVEN

1. a. Facilitate the quality of patient care
   b. Ensure documentation of progress with regard to patient-focused outcomes
   c. Facilitate interdisciplinary consistency and communication of treatment goals and progress

2. ___C___ Assessment

   ___A___ Problem identification

   ___A___ Planning

   __B, D__ Implementation

   __A, B__ Evaluation

3. (a) staff communication; (b) legal documentation; (c) evaluation; (d) accreditation; (e) training and supervision; (f) reimbursement; (g) relationship monitoring.

4. JCAHO standards mandate that the medical record shall contain the following elements of nursing care data: (a) patient assessment; (b) nursing diagnosis and/or patient needs; (c) nursing interventions; (d) patient outcomes.

5. In documenting for reimbursement, five factors need to be included: the when, where, how, what, and who of services.

6. Two ways in which the plan of care can be used for supervision are in the identification of employees' abilities, and identifying the need for further supervision, training, or education

7. The best way to ensure clarity of the progress notes is to use descriptive/observational statements.

8. For example: a. Mr. Jones refused his bath and did not want to get out of bed this morning.
   b. Miss Smith told me I was the only nurse who listened to her and wanted me to let her skip her medication and not tell the doctor.
   c. Mrs. Wharton said she was tired of taking her medicine and threw the cup across the room this morning.
   d. Mr. Bemish did not want to go to bed and cursed when I went in to obtain his admitting information.

9. a. Contain undefined periods of time
   b. Undefined quantities

c. Qualities

d. Fail to specify any objective basis for the judgment made

10. Types of data which are important to record in the progress note are: unsettled or unclear problems which need to be dealt with; noteworthy incidents or interviews; other pertinent data, such as phone calls, home visits, and family interactions; additional critical incident data; care or observations not recorded elsewhere.

11. Five additional factors which can enhance accurate communication are: correct grammar, correct spelling, legible writing, use of nonerasible ink, avoidance of repetition of data, avoidance of abbreviations, brevity.

12. Draw a line through the error, write "error," and initial.

13. Three charting formats are: block; POMR; FOCUS®; Narrative—time.

14. Vignette—The SOAP/SOAPIER format requires that chart entries be tied to a problem. In reviewing this vignette, you might choose to address the problem of pain.

SOAP: Problem #1 (Pain)

S: Constant low backache, "I need medication for pain now."

O: Restless; teary-eyed with contractions, not using breathing/relaxation techniques; anxious that husband/physician have not arrived. Strong contractions 4–5 minutes apart, lasting 40 seconds, cervix dilated 5 cm.

A: Perception of pain heightened by tension and anxiety.

P: Assist Sally to regain control, reduce pain.

I: Oriented to surroundings. Positioned for comfort, back massaged. Encouraged to use breathing/relaxation techniques with contractions. Discussed concerns, verified that someone would stay with her as she desires/needs. Arranged for contact with her mother.

E: Appears relaxed, resting quietly.

R: Reassess in 15 minutes.

The FOCUS® format provides for chart entries to be tied to a problem sign/symptom, event, or specific standard of care. Therefore, an initial entry addressing Sally's admission is acceptable, or you could choose to address the problem of pain.

FOCUS®: Admission

D: Complaining of constant low backache—requesting medication now. Restless, teary-eyed with contractions, not using breathing/relaxation techniques. Appears anxious that husband/physician have not yet arrived. Strong contractions 4–5 minutes apart, lasting 40 seconds. Cervix dilated 5 cm.

A: Oriented to surroundings. Positioned for comfort, back massaged. Encouraged to use breathing/relaxation techniques with contractions. Discussed concerns, verified someone would stay with her as she desires/needs. Arranged for Sally to call her mother. Will reassess in 15 minutes.

R: Appears relaxed, resting quietly. Will call nurse as she needs.

KEY TO COMPREHENSIVE WORK PAGE

6/28 Patient Diagnostic Statement (Nursing Diagnosis)

Skin Integrity, impaired, related to pressure, altered metabolic state, circulatory impairment, and decreased sensation evidenced by draining wound L foot.

Desired Outcomes: Patient Will

Demonstrate correction of metabolic state as evidenced by blood sugar within normal limits within (timeframe).
Be free of purulent drainage within (timeframe).
Display signs of healing by (timeframe).

INTERVENTIONS

Obtain culture of wound drainage on admission.
Administer dicloxacillin 500 mg po q 6 h starting 10 PM.
Observe for signs of hypersensitivity, that is, pruritis, urticaria, rash.
Soak foot in room temperature sterile water with betadine solution t.i.d. X15 min.
Dress wound with dry sterile dressing; use paper tape.
Administer 15 u NPH insulin s.c. q AM after daily lab (FBS) drawn.

6/28 Patient Diagnostic Statement (Nursing Diagnosis)

Pain related to physical agent (wound L foot) evidenced by verbal complaint of discomfort and guarding behavior.

Desired Outcomes: Patient Will

Report pain is minimized/relieved within (timeframe).
Ambulate normally, full weight bearing, by (timeframe).

INTERVENTIONS

Determine pain characteristics through patient's description.
Place foot cradle on bed/encourage use of loose-fitting slipper, when up.
Administer Darvon 65 mg po q4h as needed. Document effectiveness.

6/28 Patient Diagnostic Statement (Nursing Diagnosis)

Tissue Perfusion, altered: peripheral, related to decreased arterial flow evidenced by decreased pulses, pale/cool feet, thick brittle nails, numbness/tingling of feet "when walks a lot."

Desired Outcomes: Patient Will

Verbalize understanding of relationship between chronic disease (diabetes mellitus) and circulatory changes within (timeframe).

Demonstrate awareness of safety factors/proper foot care within (timeframe).

INTERVENTIONS

Elevate feet when up in chair. Avoid long periods with feet dependent.

Assess for signs of dehydration.

Monitor I/O. Encourage oral fluids.

Instruct patient to avoid constricting clothing/socks and ill-fitting shoes.

Reinforce safety precautions regarding use of heating pads, hot water bottles/soaks.

Discuss complications of disease that result in vascular changes, that is, ulceration, gangrene, muscle or bony structure changes.

Review proper foot care as outlined in teaching plan.

6/28 Patient Diagnostic Statement (Nursing Diagnosis)

Knowledge deficit: diabetic care, related to misinterpretation of information and/or lack of recall evidenced by inaccurate follow-through of instructions regarding home glucose monitoring and foot care, and failure to recognize signs/symptoms of hyperglycemia.

Desired Outcome: Patient Will

Verbalize basic understanding of disease process and treatment within (timeframe).

Perform procedure of home glucose monitoring and insulin administration correctly by (timeframe).

INTERVENTIONS

Determine patient's level of knowledge, priorities of learning needs, and desire/need for including wife in instruction.

Review factors related to/altering diabetes control, for example, stress, illness, exercise.

Review signs/symptoms of hyperglycemia, discuss prevention and evaluation of situation and when to seek medical care.

Review and provide information about routine examination of feet.

Instruct regarding prescribed insulin therapy.

Demonstrate, then observe patient in: drawing insulin into syringe, reading syringe markings, and administering dose. Assess for accuracy.

Instruct in signs/symptoms of insulin reaction/hypoglycemia.

Review "Sick Day Rules."

Recommend patient maintain record of fingerstick testing, insulin dosage/site, unusual physiologic response, dietary intake.

Refer to dietician for revision of diet.

Glossary

ANALYSIS: the process of examining and categorizing information to reach a conclusion about a patient's needs.

ASSESSMENT: the first step of the Nursing Process, during which data are collected.

BASE-LINE ASSESSMENT: initial data collection done at the time of admission/beginning of shift, and so on, with which future assessments are compared.

CHARTING: the written record of relevant details of the care given to a patient and the patient's response, including observations and changes in the patient's condition.

COLLABORATIVE PROBLEM: a need identified by another discipline that will contain a nursing component requiring nursing intervention and/or monitoring.

CUE(S): a signal that indicates a possible need/direction for care.

DAR: format for charting—data, actions, response (called FOCUS® Charting).

DEFINING CHARACTERISTICS: clinical criteria that represent the presence of a diagnostic category; cluster of signs and symptoms indicating a specific nursing diagnosis.

DIAGNOSIS: identification of a disease/condition or human response by a scientific evaluation of signs/symptoms, history, and diagnostic studies.

DIAGNOSTIC ERROR: a mistaken assumption leading to a wrong conclusion.

DIAGNOSTIC REASONING: process of problem identification used during the second step of the Nursing Process: problem sensing, rule-out process, synthesizing the data, evaluation or confirming the hypothesis, listing patient problems/needs.

ETIOLOGY: identified causes and/or contributing factors responsible for the presence of a specific patient problem/need.

EVALUATION: the fifth step of the Nursing Process during which the patient's movement toward specified outcomes is determined and the plan of care is modified or care is terminated depending on the findings.

FOCUS ASSESSMENT: gathering of data narrowed to a specific area/topic.

GOALS: broad guidelines indicating the overall direction for movement as a result of the interventions of the healthcare team; divided into long-term goals and short-term goals.

IMPLEMENT/IMPLEMENTATION: the fourth step of the Nursing Process in which the plan of care is put into action; performing identified interventions/activities.

INFER: to conclude/deduce from evidence presented.

INTUITION: a sense of something that is not clearly evidenced by known facts.

JCAHO: Joint Commission on Accreditation of Healthcare Organizations; surveying body which certifies clinical and organization performance of an institution following established guidelines.

LONG-TERM GOALS: those goals that may not be achieved prior to discharge from care but require continued attention by patient and/or others as indicated.

MEASURABLE VERB: an action/behavior which can be quantified by specific amounts of time or measure and can be seen or heard.

MEDICAL DIAGNOSIS: illnesses/conditions for which treatment is directed by a licensed physician; medical diagnoses focus on correction/prevention of the pathology of specific organs/body systems.

NANDA: North American Nursing Diagnosis Association, international group responsible for the development of nursing diagnoses.

NURSE/PATIENT RELATIONSHIP: a therapeutic relationship built on a series of interactions, developing over time, and meeting the needs of the patient.

NURSING AUDIT: procedure to evaluate the quality of nursing care provided, using established criteria/standards. Concurrent audit is done while nursing care is being performed. Retrospective audit is done after the patient is discharged from care.

NURSING DIAGNOSIS: *noun:* a label approved by NANDA identifying specific patient problems/needs. The means of describing health problems amenable to treatment by nurses; may be physical, sociologic, or psychologic. *Verb:* process of identifying specific patient problems/needs, used by some as the title of the second step of the nursing process.

NURSING INTERVENTIONS: prescriptions for specific behaviors expected for the patient, and/or actions to be carried out by nurses to promote, maintain, or restore health.

NURSING PROCESS: an orderly, logical five-step problem-solving approach for administering nursing care. Composed of assessment, problem identification, planning, implementation, and evaluation.

NURSING STANDARD: identified criterion against which nursing care is compared and evaluated; generally reflects the minimum level for nursing care.

OBJECTIVE DATA: what can be observed, for example, vital signs, behaviors, diagnostic studies.

OUTCOME: the result of actions undertaken to achieve a broader goal; measurable steps to achieve the goals of treatment and to meet discharge criteria.

PATIENT DATABASE: the compilation of data collected about a patient; it consists of the nursing history, physical examination, and results of the diagnostic studies.

PATIENT DIAGNOSTIC STATEMENT: the outcome of the diagnostic reasoning process; a three-part statement identifying the patient's problem/need, etiology of the problem/need, and the associated signs/symptoms.

P E S: format for combining a patient problem label, etiology, and signs/symptoms to create an individualized diagnostic statement.

PLANNING: the third step of the Nursing Process during which goals/outcomes are determined and interventions chosen.

PLAN OF CARE: written evidence of the second and third steps of the Nursing Process that identifies the patient's problems/needs, goals/outcomes of care, and interventions to treat the problems/needs.

POMR OR PORS: Problem-Oriented Medical Record—a method of recording data about the health status of the patient.

POTENTIAL/HIGH RISK NURSING DIAGNOSIS: a problem that may occur/recur particularly if intervention is not undertaken. As it has not yet occurred, there are no signs/symptoms when writing the patient diagnostic statement; instead, risk factors are identified.

PROBLEM IDENTIFICATION: the second step of the Nursing Process in which the data collected are analyzed and, through the process of diagnostic reasoning, specific patient diagnostic statements are created.

PROTOCOL: written guidelines of steps to be taken for providing patient care in a particular situation/condition.

RELATED FACTOR: the condition or situation which appears to demonstrate some type of patterned relationship with a specific nursing diagnosis; forms the *related to* component of the patient diagnostic statement.

RISK FACTOR: the condition or situation that may lead to the development/recurrence of a patient problem/specific nursing diagnosis.

SHORT-TERM GOALS: those goals that usually must be met prior to discharge or movement to a less acute level of care.

SOAP: format for documentation—subjective, objective, analysis, plan.

SOAPIER: format for documentation—subjective, objective, analysis, plan, implementation, evaluation, revision.

SIGN: objective or observable evidence or manifestation of a health problem.

SUBJECTIVE DATA: what the patient reports, believes, or feels.

SYMPTOM: subjectively perceptible change in the body or its functions that indicates disease or the kind or phases of disease.

SYNTHESIZE: viewing all data as a whole to provide a comprehensive picture of the patient.

VALIDATION: the process of assuring that data are factual.

WELLNESS: a state of optimal health, physical and psychosocial.

Bibliography

Anatomy, Physiology, and Pathophysiology

Carrieri, VK, et al: Pathophysiological Phenomena in Nursing: Human Response to Illness. WB Saunders, Philadelphia, 1986.

Guyton, AC: Textbook of Medical Physiology, ed. 7. WB Saunders, Philadelphia, 1987.

Hole, JW, Jr.: Human Anatomy and Physiology, ed 4. WC Brown, Dubuque, IA, 1987.

Porth, C.: Pathophysiology: Concepts of Altered Health States, ed 2. JB Lippincott, Philadelphia, 1986.

Price, SA and Wilson, LM: Pathophysiology: Clinical Concepts of Disease Processes, ed 3. McGraw-Hill, New York, 1986.

Thibodeau, GA: Anatomy and Physiology. CV Mosby, St. Louis, 1987.

Tortora, GJ and Anagnostakos, NP: Principles of Anatomy and Physiology, ed 5. Harper & Row, New York, 1986.

Community Health Nursing

Clemen-Stone, S, et al: Comprehensive Family and Community Health Nursing, ed 2. McGraw-Hill, New York, 1987.

Jarvis, LL: Community Health Nursing: Keeping the Public Healthy, ed 2. FA Davis, Philadelphia, 1985.

Logan, BB and Dawkins, CE: Family-Centered Nursing in the Community. Addison-Wesley, Menlo Park, CA, 1986.

Pender, NJ: Health Promotion in Nursing Practice, ed 2. Appleton & Lange, Norwalk, CT, 1987.

Stanhope, M and Lancaster, J: Community Health Nursing: Process and Practice for Promoting Health, ed 2. CV Mosby, St. Louis, 1988.

Critical Care Nursing

Alspach, JG and Williams, SM: Core Curriculum for Critical Care Nursing, ed 3. WB Saunders, Philadelphia, 1985.

Dolan, JT: Critical Care Nursing: Clinical Management through the Nursing Process. FA Davis, Philadelphia, in preparation.

Holloway, NM: Nursing the Critically Ill Adult, ed 3. Addison-Wesley, Menlo Park, CA, 1988.

Hudak, CM, et al: Critical Care Nursing: A Holistic Approach, ed 4. JB Lippincott, Philadelphia, 1986.

Kenner, CV, et al: Critical Care Nursing: Body, Mind, Spirit, ed 2. Little, Brown, Boston, 1985.

Moorhouse, MF, et al: Critical Care Plans: Guidelines for Patient Care. FA Davis, Philadelphia, 1987.

Fundamentals of Nursing

Kozier, B and Erb, G: Fundamentals of Nursing: Concepts and Procedures, ed 3. Addison-Wesley, Menlo Park, CA, 1987.

Kozier, B and Erb, G: Techniques in Clinical Nursing: A Nursing Process Approach. Addison-Wesley, Menlo Park, CA, 1987.

Perry, AG and Potter, PA: Clinical Nursing Skills and Techniques: Basic, Intermediate, and Advanced. CV Mosby, St. Louis, 1986.

Potter, PA and Perry, AG: Basic Nursing: Theory and Practice, CV Mosby, St. Louis, 1987.

Potter, PA and Perry, AG: Fundamentals of Nursing: Concepts, Process, and Practice, ed 2. CV Mosby, St. Louis, 1989.

Sorensen, KC and Luckmann, J: Basic Nursing: A Psychophysiologic Approach, ed 2. WB Saunders, Philadelphia, 1986.

Health Assessment

Bates, B: A Guide to Physical Examination and History Taking, ed 4. JB Lippincott, Philadelphia, 1987.

Bowers, AC and Thompson, JM: Clinical Manual of Health Assessment, ed 3. CV Mosby, St. Louis, 1988.

Malasanos, L, et al: Health Assessment, ed 3. CV Mosby, St. Louis, 1986.

Seidel, HM, et al: Mosby's Guide to Physical Examination. CV Mosby, St. Louis, 1987.

Maternity Nursing

Bobak, IM and Jensen, MD: Essentials of Maternity Nursing: The Nurse and the Child-bearing Family, ed 2. CV Mosby, St. Louis, 1987.

Doenges, ME, et al: Maternal/Newborn Care Plans: Guidelines for Client Care. FA Davis, Philadelphia, 1988.

Malinowski, JS: Nursing Care during the Labor Process, ed 3. FA Davis, Philadelphia, 1989.

Neeson, JD: Clinical Manual of Maternity Nursing. JB Lippincott, Philadelphia, 1987.

Neeson, JD and May, KA: Comprehensive Maternity Nursing. JB Lippincott, Philadelphia, 1986.

Olds, SB, et al: Maternal-Newborn Nursing: A Family-Centered Approach, ed 3. Addison-Wesley, Menlo Park, CA, 1988.

Reeder, SJ, et al: Maternity Nursing, ed 16. JB Lippincott, Philadelphia, 1987.

Medical-Surgical Nursing

Brunner, LS and Suddarth, DS: Textbook of Medical-Surgical Nursing, ed 6. JB Lippincott, Philadelphia, 1988.

Cella, JH and Watson, J: Nurse's Manual of Laboratory Tests. FA Davis, Philadelphia, 1989.

Fischbach, FT: A Manual of Laboratory Diagnostic Tests, ed 3. JB Lippincott, Philadelphia, 1988.

Kneisl, CR and Ames, SW: Adult Health Nursing: A Biopsychosocial Approach. Addison-Wesley, Menlo Park, CA, 1986.

Lewis, S: Medical-Surgical Nursing: Assessment and Management of Clinical Problems, ed 2. McGraw-Hill, New York, 1987.

Luckmann, J and Sorensen, KC: Medical-Surgical Nursing: A Psychophysiologic Approach, ed 3. WB Saunders, Philadelphia, 1987.

Patrick, ML, et al: Medical-Surgical Nursing: Pathophysiological Concepts. JB Lippincott, Philadelphia, 1986.

Phipps, WJ, et al: Medical-Surgical Nursing: Concepts and Clinical Practice, ed 3. CV Mosby, St. Louis, 1986.

Nursing Process/Nursing Diagnoses

Alfaro, RA: Application of Nursing Process: A Step-by-Step Guide to Care Planning, ed 2. JB Lippincott, Philadelphia, 1990.

American Nurses Association: Nursing: A social policy statement. Pub Code: NP-63 3SM 12/80, Kansas City, 1980.

American Nurses Association: Standards of nursing practice. Pub Code: NO41 10M 1:77, Kansas City, 1973.

Atkinson, LD and Murray, ME: Understanding the Nursing Process, ed 3. Macmillan, New York, 1986.

Benjamin, A: The Helping Interview, ed 3. Houghton Mifflin, Boston, 1981.

Brunckhorst, L, et al: Who's using nursing diagnoses? AJN, February, 1989: 267–268.

Bulechek, GM and McCloskey, JC: Nursing Interventions: Treatments for Nursing Diagnoses. WB Saunders, Philadelphia, 1985.

Carpenito, LB: Handbook of Nursing Diagnosis 1989–90. JB Lippincott, Philadelphia, 1989.

Carpenito, LB: Nursing Diagnosis: Application to Clinical Practice, ed 2. JB Lippincott, Philadelphia, 1987.

Documentation. Nursing 88 Books. Springhouse, Springhouse, PA, 1988.

Doenges, ME and Moorhouse, MF: Nurse's Pocket Guide: Nursing Diagnoses with Interventions, ed 3. FA Davis, Philadelphia, 1990.

Doenges, ME, et al: Nursing Care Plans: Guidelines for Planning Patient Care, ed 2. FA Davis, Philadelphia, 1989.

Dolan, M: Why nurses & doctors should be partners in diagnosis. Nursing 90 20(11):41, 1990.

Eggland, ET: Charting: How and why to document your care daily—and fully. Nursing 88 18(11):76–84, 1988.

Gettrust, KV: Applied Nursing Diagnosis: Guides for Comprehensive Care Planning. John Wiley, New York, 1985.

Gordon, M: Manual of Nursing Diagnosis 1988–1989. CV Mosby, St. Louis, 1989.

Gordon, M: Nursing Diagnosis: Process and Application, ed 2. McGraw-Hill, New York, 1987.

Hanson, P: Focus charting—A new documentation tool. Coordinator, March 1986: 25–27.

Iyer, PW: New trends in charting. Nursing 91, January, 1991: 48–50.

Iyer, PW, et al: Nursing Process and Nursing Diagnosis. WB Saunders, Philadelphia, 1986.

Kettenbach, G: Writing S.O.A.P. Notes. FA Davis, Philadelphia, 1990.

Kim, MJ, et al: Pocket Guide to Nursing Diagnoses, ed 3. CV Mosby, St. Louis, 1989.

Lampe, SS: Focus® Charting: Creative Nursing Management, ed 4. Minneapolis, MN, 1988.

Lampe, SS: Focus charting: Streamlining documentation. Nursing Management 16(7):43–46, 1985.

Leuner, JD, et al: Mastering the Nursing Process: A Case Method Approach. FA Davis, Philadelphia, 1990.

Little, DE and Carnevali, DL: Nursing Care Planning, ed 2. JB Lippincott, Philadelphia, 1976.

McCabe, BW: Evaluating the use of a focused data collection tool for the generation of nursing diagnoses: A replication study. Clinical Judgment and Decision-Making: The Future with Nursing Diagnosis. John Wiley, New York, 1987: 141–143.

McFarland, GK and McFarlane, EA: Nursing Diagnosis & Intervention. CV Mosby, St. Louis, 1989.

McHugh, MK, ed: Nursing Process. HNP 1:3. Aspen, May, 1987.

Maslow, A: Toward a Psychology of Being. Van Nostrand, New York, 1968.

Moorhouse, M and Doenges, M: Nurse's Clinical Pocket Manual. FA Davis, Philadelphia, 1990.

Nightingale, F: Notes on Nursing. Harrison, St. Martin's Lane, London WC, 1859.

Patient Teaching. Nursing 87 Books. Springhouse, Springhouse, PA, 1987.

Radwin, LE: Research on diagnostic reasoning in nursing. Nursing Diagnosis 1(2): 70–77. April/June, 1990.

Rew, L: Nursing intuition, too powerful—and too valuable—to ignore. Nursing 87. July, 1987: 43–45.

Richard, J: Walking rounds: A step in the right direction. Nursing 89 19(6): 63–64.

Samhammer, JH and Larson, K: Interacting with Patients. Macmillan, New York, 1963.

Shore, LS: Nursing Diagnosis: What It Is and How to Do It, a Programmed Text. Medical College of Virginia Hospitals, Richmond, 1988.

Svanda, C: Two ways to sharpen your charting skills: Key words show what's important. RN. December, 1986: 32–33.

Ulrich, S, et al: Nursing Care Planning Guides: A Nursing Diagnosis Approach. WB Saunders, Philadelphia, 1986.

Nutrition

Dudek, SG: Nutrition Handbook for Nursing Practice. JB Lippincott, Philadelphia, 1987.

Lewis, CM: Nutrition and Nutritional Therapy in Nursing. Appleton & Lange, Norwalk, CT, 1985.

Robinson, CH: Normal and Therapeutic Nutrition, ed 17. MacMillan, New York, 1986.

Stanfield, P and Hui, YH: Nutrition and Diet Therapy: Self-Instruction Modules. Jones & Bartlett, Boston, 1986.

Pediatric Nursing

Foster, RLR, et al: Family-Centered Nursing Care of Children. WB Saunders, Philadelphia, 1989.

James, SR: Child Health Nursing: Essential Care of Children and Families. Addison-Wesley, Menlo Park, CA, 1988.

Marlow, DR and Redding, BA: Textbook of Pediatric Nursing, ed 6. WB Saunders, Philadelphia, 1988.

Mott, SR, et al: Nursing Care of Children and Families: A Holistic Approach. Addison-Wesley, Menlo Park, CA, 1985.

Whaley, LF and Wong, DL: Essentials of Pediatric Nursing, ed 3. CV Mosby, St. Louis, 1988.

Whaley, LF and Wong, DL: Nursing Care of Infants and Children, ed 3. CV Mosby, St. Louis, 1986.

Pharmacology

Baer, C and Williams, B: Clinical Pharmacology and Nursing. Springhouse, Springhouse, PA, 1988.

Clark, JB, et al: Pharmacological Basis of Nursing Practice, ed 2. CV Mosby, St. Louis, 1986.

Deglin, JH and Vallerand, AH: Davis's Drug Guide for Nurses. FA Davis, Philadelphia, 1988.

Govoni, L and Hayes, J: Drugs and Nursing Implications, ed 6. Appleton & Lange, Norwalk, CT, 1988.

Malseed, RT and Harrigan, GS: Textbook of Pharmacology and Nursing Care: Using the Nursing Process. JB Lippincott, Philadelphia, 1989.

Mathewson, MK: Pharmacotherapeutics: A Nursing Process Approach. FA Davis, Philadelphia, 1986.

McHenry, LM and Salerno, E: Mosby's Pharmacology in Nursing, ed 17. CV Mosby, St. Louis, 1989.

Shlafer, M and Marieb, EN: The Nurse, Pharmacology, and Drug Therapy. Addison-Wesley, Menlo Park, CA, 1989.

Spencer, RT, et al: Clinical Pharmacology and Nursing Management, ed 2. JB Lippincott, Philadelphia, 1986.

Psychiatric/Mental Health Nursing

Beck, CK, et al: Mental Health-Psychiatric Nursing: A Holistic Life-Cycle Approach, ed 2. CV Mosby, St. Louis, 1988.

Diagnostic and Statistical Manual of Mental Disorders, ed 3, revised. American Psychiatric Association, Washington, DC, 1987.

Doenges, ME, et al: Psychiatric Care Plans: Guidelines for Client Care. FA Davis, Philadelphia, 1989.

Johnson, BS: Psychiatric-Mental Health Nursing: Adaptation and Growth, ed 2. JB Lippincott, Philadelphia, 1989.

Stuart, GW and Sundeen, SJ: Principles and Practice of Psychiatric Nursing, ed 3. CV Mosby, St. Louis, 1987.

Townsend, MC: Nursing Diagnoses in Psychiatric Nursing: A Pocket Guide for Care Plan Construction. FA Davis, Philadelphia, 1988.

Wilson, HS and Kneisl, CR: Psychiatric Nursing, ed 3. Addison-Wesley, Menlo Park, CA, 1988.

Index

Numbers followed by an "f" indicate figures; numbers followed by a "t" indicate tabular material.